Hospital Mergers—
Why They Work, Why They Don't

Larry Scanlan

press

HEALTH FORUM, INC.
An American Hospital Association Company
Chicago

This publication is designed to provide accurate and authoritative information in regard to the subject matter covered. It is sold with the understanding that neither the author nor the publisher is engaged in rendering legal, accounting, or other professional services. If legal advice or other expert assistance is required, the services of a competent professional should be sought.

The views expressed in this publication are strictly those of the author and do not represent the official positions of the American Hospital Association.

Cover design by Cheri Kusek

ISBN: 978-1-55648-375-2   Item Number: 108100

Library of Congress Cataloging-in-Publication Data
Scanlan, Larry.
   Hospital mergers—why they work, why they don't / Larry Scanlan.
     p. cm.
   Includes index.
   ISBN 978-1-55648-375-2 (alk. paper)
  1. Hospital mergers—United States—Case studies. 2. Hospitals—Medical staff—Mergers—United States—Case studies. 3. Hospitals—Administration. I. Title.
   RA981.A2S27 2010
   362.11068′1—dc22   2010015219

To my wife and best friend, Connie;
and our four children and their (spouses):
Kevin (Becca), Pam, Tina (Dave), and Tricia (Jim);
and our grandchildren:
Airick, Allison, Angela, Jake, Kelley, and Shane

My thanks to our Heavenly Father and Lord Jesus
for each of them

Contents

List of Figures and Tables

About the Author

Larry Scanlan has more than thirty-five years of executive and financial health care management experience, having served the first half of his career as a hospital and health system executive and the second half as a consultant to hospitals, health systems, and academic medical centers.

Currently Mr. Scanlan is president of Insight Health Partners LLC, a consulting firm providing operational improvement and strategic services to the health care industry. In addition, he is president of his own executive coaching firm, Scanlan & Associates LLC, assisting executives to be in a better position to provide leadership to their organizations.

From the time his consulting career began in 1991, he has worked with hundreds of clients throughout the United States. He served as president of The Hunter Group from 1998 to 2002 and as managing director of Navigant Consulting's health care practice from 2002 to 2006. This experience has led him to become a trusted adviser to executives and board members in matters related to mergers, performance improvement, and strategic initiatives. Before entering the consulting field, he served as chief financial officer of a community hospital and went on to serve as chief executive officer of two hospitals.

His 2005 article on leadership, "Leading with Purpose," and his 1995 article on mergers, "Building Consensus for Integration," both won Article of the Year honors from *Healthcare Financial Management* magazine.

Mr. Scanlan is a member of the American College of Healthcare Executives and the International Coach Federation. He is also a certified public accountant and a fellow of the Healthcare Financial Management Association, having also served on its national board. In addition, he is chairman of the board of Peirce College, a private, not-for-profit four-year college in Philadelphia.

Preface

I began my first job in health care in 1973 at a Catholic hospital whose sister-leaders had decided to merge the organization with another hospital under one management team. This was an era during which little discussion about mergers took place. The two hospitals were a mere three miles apart, but the differences in their culture and attitudes made them seem as if they were 3,000 miles apart. One was a suburban hospital, the other an inner-city hospital. Debates about what services should be kept open seemed endless, as was the decision making on where to prioritize capital investment. The inner-city hospital was losing money; the suburban hospital personnel resented "carrying" the inner-city hospital. I found the entire experience fascinating.

As my career progressed with different employers, I found the subject of mergers, acquisitions, and selling or leasing hospitals increasingly prevalent in senior management and board discussions in the context of strategic direction and what was best for the organization. In one professional role, I worked as chief financial officer for a for-profit hospital company on the East Coast that later merged with a hospital company on the West Coast. Working on the for-profit side of the hospital industry was valuable to my career progress, and the merger proved to be yet another interesting experience. Neither company is around today, a fact that represents the inherent risk in merger activity.

Later, I accepted the role of president of a not-for-profit hospital that had recently merged. This was the mid-1980s, and the concept of "health systems" was starting to take hold. The merger seemed to make sense, but as I began my new job, I learned the merger was put together quickly by four board members from each organization with the help of the CEOs. Next I discovered that the physicians of both hospitals did not support the merger, in large part because they were not involved in its planning.

If that were not enough, the Federal Trade Commission launched an investigation into the merger. It also became apparent that the merger was part of a defensive strategy for the larger organization; it lacked an "offensive" strategy with no real plan to invest and grow services at the smaller facility. The federal investigation became a convenient excuse to break up a newly formed system that was already struggling. The organization then experienced "de-merging," a costly learning experience unto itself. Moreover, we needed to find another strategic partner. My fascination for hospital mergers—why they work and why they don't—was just beginning, and I was learning my own lessons on what steps and tasks I would perform differently the next time around, assuming there was a next time.

In the second half of my career I joined a fledgling health care firm that would go on to develop a prominent name as a national hospital consulting company. My nationwide exposure to mergers was greatly expanded, as often we were called upon to "fix" mergers that were not working. We later converted this experience into helping organizations better think through merger strategies at the beginning of the process. My interest in this subject led me to write an article in 1995 about the merger process, which won an award for best article of the year from *Healthcare Financial Management* magazine.

During my years as president of The Hunter Group and later as managing director of Navigant Consulting's health care practice, I had the privilege to work with many organizations throughout the country on merger-related matters. Working behind the scenes and gaining insight into why these strategies worked or failed was intriguing. I decided it was time to write a book about the subject to flesh out the reasons for the mixed track record mergers have in hospitals and, frankly, almost any other industry.

In chapter 1, we describe the historical context of merger activity of the last several decades, as the strategy of mergers has affected many hospitals and the communities they serve. Mergers in the hospital industry were a rare transaction until the 1990s.

Chapter 2 considers the reason to merge. Without sound reasons to engage in merger activity, the prospects of strategic success are diminished, as critical understanding of the reasons to explore a merger is necessary to reach consensus among management and the board and, eventually, other critical constituents, such as physicians, employees, and the community at large.

In chapter 3, we examine the process of merging—the "how do we go about this?" question. Merger considerations require significant time and financial investment to go through the process and come away with the maximum opportunity for success. Taking shortcuts, as I learned in one of my hospital chief executive jobs, is costly, in more ways than you may even think.

The impact of culture on mergers is discussed in chapter 4. Issues surrounding organizational culture are considered a "soft" component of mergers, but because they can make or break a merger, to understand and resolve them is critical for even the most logical of mergers to work. We review a number of cases related to culture issues—we have no shortage of them available to consider—and reveal how others have dealt with them.

Chapter 5 explores the impact of leadership on hospital and health system mergers. It seems many mergers come down to deciding who will serve as CEO, and even assuming an organization can resolve this question, it must address issues related to forming the new board, including who will serve as the first board chair. Next, decisions must be made about who will be on the senior management team, yet another critical hurdle that must be successfully negotiated.

In chapter 6, we discuss the outcomes of mergers and focus most of our attention on determining those factors that allowed mergers to succeed and that particularly represented gains for patient care and the community.

The question of whether the unprecedented merger activity of the last fifteen years is likely to continue is considered in chapter 7. Will mergers continue to be considered in most organizations' strategic planning? We attempt to peek into the future and make some judgments about the likelihood of merger-like activity over the next decade.

Certainly, leaders experience both success and failure in any job. Our shortcomings are temporary as long as we assess and learn from our disappointments. Our victories are milestones that energize us and carry us through a journey that will entail yet more disappointments—and, we hope, even more successes—as we learn how to lead and manage along the ups and downs of the leadership journey.

The purpose in writing this book is to lend an understanding of the lessons to be learned from our review of hospital mergers and the experiences of those who participated in them and apply these lessons to the current strategic challenges and opportunities organizations face today.

The objective is for the material to be instructive and educational for current and future health care leaders, including trustees, educators, and health administration students.

I thank all the executives who shared their experiences, providing teaching moments for readers to take forward.

Acknowledgments

The thought and dream of writing a book, perhaps making a contribution to a profession I have enjoyed working in for more than thirty-five years, had been on my mind for several years. Moving from concept to actual research began in late 2008. But like most significant undertakings, it is only possible to complete such work with the help, understanding, and support of other people. I am blessed to have had such support.

First, I had the support of my wife, Connie. She possesses in her character the gift of encouragement, truly, I believe, a God-given talent. We need more people with this gift. Not only did she encourage me to go ahead with "the book project" but she also was the first reviewer of each chapter written. Having spent her career as an administrative assistant to CEOs of industry, education, and health care, she always wanted to be an English teacher. Well, she got a chance to fulfill that desire, at least in part, while critiquing renditions of each chapter in a project that took more than a year to complete. She would have been a fine English teacher.

I am deeply appreciative of several other special people who invested considerable time in this endeavor. Kathy Kronenberg is the chief operating officer of Insight Health Partners, a hospital consulting firm. I met Kathy in 1991 when she was working for a client of mine in El Paso, Texas. I always said if I had the chance to hire her, I would, and that chance came later in the decade when she became part of a firm I was working with. Her background in health planning, managed care, business development, and administrative organization, as well as her ability to pay attention to detail while understanding the big picture, is an exceptional combination of skills that few possess. She was my right-hand person when I managed and led The Hunter Group and, later, the health care practice division of Navigant Consulting. She volunteered to review this manuscript from the perspective of her professional experience working with many hospitals, including those involved in merger projects. Her critique throughout the process has proved invaluable, and I am indebted to her for giving up such time.

Becky Rust, who has been my administrative assistant for many years, made a significant investment in this project. Becky is the most professional and experienced executive assistant I have encountered in my career. We met in the early 1990s when she was the assistant to a health care system chief executive. Having spent many years in health care, she understands the industry and is able to make sound suggestions in terms of content and how that content gets expressed in writing; as an added bonus, she is one of the few people who can read my handwriting and translate it into a typed document. Besides this unique talent, she is incredibly quick, works all hours of day or night to complete a project, and makes sure it is done exactly right. There simply is no one else like her. Her professionalism and diligence significantly helped bring this book to fruition.

I would also like to thank a group of executives whose constructive comments and encouragement for the rationale of this book were helpful in bringing it to reality: Rodney Hochman, MD, CEO of Swedish Medical Center; William Kerr, retired CEO of the University of California, San Francisco Medical Center; Beth O'Brien, RN, senior vice president of Operations and group executive officer of Catholic Health Initiatives; P. Terrence O'Rourke, MD, executive vice president and chief clinical officer of Trinity Health; and Robert V. Stanek, recently (at the time of this writing) retired CEO of Catholic Health East.

I would like to recognize two other people, whom I consider friends. My thanks to Jeff Brown of FTI Consulting for his assistance in the interview process. Jeff introduced me to a number of people who shared their real-life accounts of merger activity within their organizations.

I also would like to acknowledge Joe Chavlovich of Insight Health Partners for his constructive assistance in selected portions of the manuscript. Joe is one of the best financial executives I have ever met and had the privilege to work with.

My special thanks also to the more than sixty hospital and health system executives, trustees, doctors and nurses, and consultants who took time from their busy schedules to speak with me about their observations and experiences on the subject of hospital mergers. It was indeed my privilege to listen to and gain knowledge from what they had to offer through their considerable and valuable insight.

My most sincere appreciation to American Hospital Association's Health Forum, Inc., for its decision to take on this project. My thanks to Richard Hill, MA, MMgt., editorial director of AHA Press, for his assistance, communication, and feedback during the process. My thanks also to Joyce Dunne, contract project manager for AHA Press, for her help and excellent work on the manuscript. Rick, Joyce, and the Health Forum team have been a pleasure to work with over this past year. Thank you for your confidence.

In two decades of consulting, having had the opportunity to travel extensively throughout the United States meeting and working with many fine executives and clinicians has been the best part of my work. I learned much, and I always tried to give each client my very best effort and advice. The lessons from my own interactions with these clients are expressed throughout the book. I have great respect for their administrative and clinical leadership, and it has been my privilege to have been involved with such outstanding people over the years. Their jobs are challenging, and their professional contribution to their respective organizations and to the communities they serve has my deepest respect. I thank every executive, doctor, nurse, manager, health care worker, and trustee whom I have had the opportunity to meet and who made my career a special memory I will always cherish. You are part of this story.

Hospital Mergers—
Why They Work, Why They Don't

1

Merger Mania:
Recent History

Hospital merger mania—before 1994 we hardly noticed such activity, and few people discussed it. In fact, the American Hospital Association was the only organization to track mergers prior to 1994. Between 1990 and 1993, the average annual number of hospital mergers was seventeen;[1] starting in 1994 and up until the present time, however, hospital mergers have become a strategic option that most health system executives and their boards need to consider at one time or another. During the last fifteen years, well over a thousand community hospital mergers took place. Add to this statistic the mergers or formations of multistate regional and national systems during this same time, and it is apparent that the influence of mergers and acquisitions has touched most hospitals and markets in the United States. In the context of this book the word *merger* is the umbrella term that marks a change of control, whether it is a true legal merger, an acquisition, a joint operating agreement, a long-term lease, or a comprehensive joint venture as defined in figure 1-1.

The apex of hospital merger activity was a five-year period between 1994 and 1998, when an average of about 150 community hospital mergers took place each year. More hospital merger transactions took place during this five-year period than in the ensuing ten years, from 1999 to 2008,[2] as seen in table 1-1.

Furthermore, in 2009, the most recent year of available data, the number of deals and the number of facilities involved in deals indicated continued decline in hospital merger activity.[3]

Figure 1-1.   Legal Definitions of Transactions

Joint Venture	A combination of only some of the operations of two or more entities*
Affiliation	An arrangement by which two organizations remain independent but have influence on each other†
Acquisition	A legal transaction by which all or part of the ownership or assets of one organization are acquired by another†
Consolidation	In a nontechnical sense, virtually any legal transaction by which the assets and operations of two organizations are combined into one†
Merger	A corporate transaction by which two similar corporations come together permanently, leaving a single survivor†

*David A. Ettinger and Stanford P. Benenbaum, *BNA's Health Law and Business Series, Health Care Mergers and Acquisitions: The Antitrust Perspective* (Washington, DC: Bureau of National Affairs, Inc., 1996), 1400.01.C.

†American Hospital Association (AHA), *Glossary of Hospital and Health Care System Merger, Acquisition and Consolidation Terms* (Chicago: AHA, 1989), 1–4.

Table 1-1.   Approximate Number of Community Hospital Mergers or Acquisitions with Other Community Hospitals or Health Care Systems, 1994–2008

	1994–98	1999–2008	15-Year Total
Not-for-Profit or Public	457	231	688
Investor-Owned	51	101	152
NFP/Public with Investor-Owned	236	268	504
Total	**744**	**600**	**1,344**

Source: Compilation of community hospital transactions based on *Modern Healthcare's Annual Report on Mergers and Acquisitions.* Our numbers differ somewhat due to our elimination of specialty hospitals, duplicative listings between years, and elimination of announced or pending deals that appeared not to close.

Between 1994 and 1998, we saw the confluence of a number of factors relating to merger activity:

- Expectations of increased managed care contracting and pricing via capitation
- An increase in merger and acquisition activity within the investor-owned sector and resulting fear within not-for-profit organizations of aggressive takeover tactics by companies such as Columbia/HCA
- The debate on national health care coverage ("Hillary Care") led by former First Lady Hillary Clinton

Community Hospital Mergers That Worked

Mease Hospital, located in Dunedin, Florida, was the sole Mease-operated organization until the 1980s, when an administrator decided to construct a second hospital, Mease Countryside Hospital, some seven miles away in what was perceived to be a high-growth area. However, the hospital was never fully developed. The Mease board of directors considered this hospital to be an outpost, so far away (on the other side of a major north-south state highway) that it refused to even hold board meetings in this less-than-full-service hospital. If you were a nursing supervisor at Mease Countryside Hospital in the early 1990s, you found yourself without the daily on-site presence of a hospital administrator because a leader from the flagship hospital visited only two days a week.

A new administrator took over in 1992, facing both financial and medical staff challenges due to the breakup of the hospital's well-known physician clinic, Mease Clinic. He and his board chair had the courage to explore partnership or merger options early in his administration. They found a partner in what until then had been the organization's lifelong primary competitor, Morton Plant Hospital, located in Clearwater, Florida.

The two organizations created a joint venture (rather than the desired merger) out of legal necessity from a U.S. Department of Justice consent order in 1994. However, the financial backing from the joint venture with Morton Plant permitted the expansion of Mease Countryside Hospital.

Fast-forward ten years. Mease Countryside has grown from 100 beds to 350 beds. It has won seven "top 100"[4] hospital awards for patient safety over the last eleven years as it has become an important delivery system and financial engine of its current four-hospital system. Furthermore, to illustrate the changes and trends in the marketplace, at the end of the legal consent period, Mease and Morton Plant hospitals fully merged in 2005. Today, this system is considered successful. In addition to Mease's top 100 designation, Morton Plant is the only hospital to be recognized with the top 100 award in cardiovascular care in each of the eleven years the award has been given.[5,6]

On to the West Coast, in California, over the last fifteen years more merger activity has taken place than in any state in the United States; it also led the country in activity during the merger mania period of 1994 to 1998.[7] (See Appendix A for a state-by-state summary of merger activity during this period as well as the subsequent ten years.)

If you were an administrator or a finance executive at California Pacific Medical Center (CPMC) during that time, you were likely trying to bring together two hospitals, Pacific Medical Center and Children's Medical Center, in San Francisco as a subsystem of the California Health System. The medical and financial environment featured aggressive managed care companies whose pricing, capitation, and utilization review procedures resulted in decreasing hospital revenues. Serious erosion of cash threatened the viability of the San Francisco entities, and the key strategic initiative was to merge with the growing Sutter Health System in 1994.

Physician Martin Brotman, who never imagined himself as a hospital chief executive officer (CEO), took over as chief executive of CPMC in 1994. He recruited a consultant from the firm helping with the turnaround and named him chief operating officer. What was the outcome of this merger? Fifteen years later, the same leadership team is in place through the end of 2009. Four hospitals now comprise the San Francisco subsystem enterprise, which has enjoyed year after year of solid performance within the twenty-four-hospital Sutter Health.

Community Hospital Mergers That Did Not Work

If only all mergers turned out as well as the two just described. But if you were a head nurse, financial analyst, or housekeeper at Grant Hospital in Chicago, you had a different experience. In 1994, your neighborhood hospital was sold to Columbia, the for-profit health care giant that seemed to dominate other health care entities during much of the 1990s. And if you stayed employed at Grant, four years later, your hospital was sold again, this time by Columbia to Doctors Community Healthcare Corporation, headquarted in Scottsdale, Arizona. Then, incredibly, one year later, Doctors Community Healthcare Corporation sold Grant Hospital to Edgewater Medical Center in Chicago for $17.5 million. Some four years later, in 2002, Grant was sold at an auction to Merit Health of Denver. Four ownership changes in an eight-year period—the last being an auction—foreshadow the outcome for Grant: The hospital does not exist today.

Back in California, if you worked at Daniel Freeman Hospital up to the beginning of the 2000s, you were an employee of Carondelet Health System, a Catholic system based in St. Louis, Missouri. Carondelet sold Freeman Hospital in 2001 to Tenet, the large for-profit system now headquartered in Dallas. Three years later, Tenet sold Freeman to Centinela Health. Three years after this transaction, in 2007, Centinela sold Freeman to Prime Healthcare. So, your once not-for-profit hospital paycheck has now been produced by four different owners in this decade. Furthermore, the system that began this chain of sales, Carondelet, itself became part of Ascension Health in 2002. Ascension is the largest Catholic hospital system in the United States in terms of revenue,[8] with more than seventy hospitals.

Large-System Mergers and Academic Medical Centers

When it comes to large systems, it seems the formation of Ascension in 1999 from the combination of the Daughters of Charity in St. Louis and St. Joseph Health System in Michigan appears, ten years later, to be successful. Other large not-for-profit systems formed by mergers in the 1990s, such as Catholic Health Initiatives, CHRISTUS Health, and Catholic Health East, affected hundreds of hospitals and communities. Interestingly, since the formation of systems such as Ascension, Banner, and Trinity in 1999, no significant system-to-system mergers *within* the not-for-profit arena have taken place in the ensuing ten years.

Large investor-owned systems, such as Hospital Corporation of America (HCA) and Tenet, despite their own numerous challenges, have also been sustainable. Tenet, for instance, which formed from the 1995 combination of National Medical Enterprises and American Medical International, remains one of the biggest for-profit systems.

Other significant investor-owned mergers occurred in the 1990s, such as HealthTrust acquiring Epic in 1994, followed a year later by HealthTrust being acquired by Columbia/HCA. Community Health Systems acquired Hallmark Health in 1994 and continued to expand, with its most recent blockbuster acquisition being Triad in 2007. Table 1-2 illustrates multistate large-system transactions from 1994 through 1999.

Table 1-2. Significant System Mergers, 1994–99

	Investor Owned		Not-for-Profit
1994	Columbia-HCA	1994	—
	HealthTrust–Epic		
	OrNda–American Healthcare Management and Summit Health		
	Champion Healthcare Corporation–AmeriHealth		
	Community Health Systems–Hallmark Healthcare Corporation		
1995	Columbia/HCA-HealthTrust	1995	Catholic Healthcare West (CHW)–Daughters of Charity Health System West
	American Medical–National Medical Enterprises		
1996	Community Health Systems goes private	1996	Catholic Health Initiatives forms from merger of three systems
	Community Health–Dynamic Health		Catholic Health East forms from three East Coast systems
	Champion Healthcare–Paracelsus Healthcare		
	NetCare Health–Southern Health Corporation		
	Principal Hospital Company–Brim Healthcare Group		

(Continued on next page)

Table 1-2.   (Continued)

	Investor Owned		Not-for-Profit
1997	Tenet-OrNda		—
1998	—	1998	Marion Health System (Tulsa, OK) formed from four congregations
			CHW buys 8 hospitals from UniHealth
1999	Columbia sells 33 hospitals to Triad	1999	Ascension formed: Daughter of Charity National–Sisters of St. Joseph Health System
	Columbia sells 23 hospitals to LifePoint Hospitals		Banner Health System formed: Samaritan (Phoenix) and Lutheran (Fargo, ND)
	Tenet sells 10 hospitals to IASIS Healthcare		CHRISTUS Health formed: Incarnate Word Health (San Antonio)– Sisters of Charity (Houston)
			Bon Secours Health (MD) acquires 8 of the 9 hospitals owned by Franciscan Health (NY)
			Trinity formed: Mercy Health (MI)–Holy Cross Health (South Bend, IN)*

Note: Does not include specialty hospital system mergers.

*Merger announced in 1999, closed in 2000.

Source: Modern Healthcare's Annual Report on Mergers and Acquisitions, 1994–2000.

However, in larger systems, just as with community hospitals, merger actions do not always turn out well. The 1995 combination of Catholic Healthcare West and the Daughters of Charity–West, of California, split up six years later. On the investor-owned side, Quorum, the for-profit entity that owned a modest number of hospitals and managed many more during the 1990s, was bought by Triad in 2001. Triad itself was formed two years earlier when Columbia divested thirty-three hospitals. Triad began in 1999 and then, in less than ten years, as mentioned earlier, was acquired by Community Health Systems in 2007.

Hospital Corporation of America, the most substantive for-profit hospital company in operation, with 172 hospitals and 95 outpatient centers covering 21 states, was purchased by a private equity consortium in 2006.[9] The $20.9 billion price for HCA ranked it the thirty-second largest transaction of all mergers in any industry in the last decade.[10]

Academic medical centers and major teaching hospitals have also engaged in merger and alliance activity as a strategic option, having attempted to merge with each other, enter into joint ventures with investor-owned companies, or acquire community hospitals. Failures in this arena, such as the separation of the merged clinical operations of Stanford University and University of California, San Francisco and the dismantling of the Mount Sinai–New York University medical centers in 1998, have been well documented. On the other hand, mergers by Presbyterian and New York hospitals in 1998; Indiana University and Methodist hospitals, which formed Clarion Health in 1997; and Partners HealthCare, founded by Brigham and Women's and Massachusetts General hospitals in 1994 have proved sustainable to date.

As to academic and teaching hospitals partnering with the investor-owned side, Columbia/HCA's 80 percent investment in Tulane Medical Center, in New Orleans, is still intact, as is Universal Health Services' partnership with George Washington

University Hospital, in Washington, D.C.; in contrast, Hahne-mann Medical Center in Philadelphia, which sold to Tenet, later was sold to Drexel University.

The outcomes of academic medical centers folding commu-nity hospitals into their sphere are also mixed. The University of California, Los Angeles acquisition of Santa Monica Medi-cal Center in 1995 is still intact. A contrasting case is that of the Hospital of the University of Pennsylvania's acquisition of suburban Philadelphia's Phoenixville Hospital in 1997. Some seven years later, Phoenixville was sold to for-profit Commu-nity Health Systems.

Merger Considerations

Mergers in any industry are part of everyday strategic activity in the U.S. and global economies. One recent study found in excess of 300,000 mergers across the globe in the last decade—about 87 mergers a day. Many of these alliances did not result in positive outcomes; reviewing the names involved in some of the failed mergers is like walking through a corporate graveyard. The biggest U.S. merger of the last decade, Time Warner and America Online, has been undone, long known to be a failed merger.[11] Certainly, however, there are successes as well.

Hospitals in the last fifteen years have also become part of this business merger activity. Mergers may be a viable way toward a more secure future for the organization or its share-holders; however, what might start out as a rational discussion of strategic options can easily become emotional.

The people affected by a hospital merger are many: manage-ment; board members with lifelong community relationships; doctors, some who have great influence in an organization (a growing number of whom are employees); hospital employ-ees; volunteers; fund-raising foundations; shareholders for the investor-owned enterprises; community leaders; banks and bondholders of hospital debt; and most importantly, the community—*patients*. Will the people for whom our hospitals exist, the patients, be better off with a merger in terms of access, improved cost structures, and better technology and facilities?

These are important considerations for any community or region, given the fact that health care, as a percentage of the U.S. gross national product, exceeds 17 percent,[12] and 30 cents of every health care dollar is spent on hospital care[13]—the largest portion of the health care distribution pie. Furthermore, hospitals are often one of the largest employers in a community or city, sometimes *the* largest employer. Thus, contemplation of a merger may portend economic consequences and certainly engenders political debate among board members, community leaders, and elected officials. Of the approximately 4,900 hospitals in the United States, less than 900 are for-profit; the remainder are not-for-profit, tax-exempt hospitals (about 3,000) or local district or state-owned public hospitals (about 1,100).[14]

During the merger mania period of 1994 to 1998, approximately 744 community hospital mergers occurred, more than 60 percent of which involved the merger of not-for-profit entities with either other not-for-profits or publicly owned hospitals such as district hospitals (see table 1-1).

In the ensuing ten years (1999 to 2008), nearly half of the mergers involved transactions between not-for-profits and investor-owned (for-profit) entities, as the ability to swap hospitals back and forth presented opportunities for both types of ownership groups. For all the angst—the not-for-profits and their associations sometimes protest the concept of being affiliated with investor-owned groups—no shortage of for-profit firms was (or is) looking to buy or sell hospitals with not-for-profits or with each other.

Figure 1-2 lists investor-owned firms that have been involved in hospital transitions over the last fifteen years. Perhaps a few

**Figure 1-2.   Investor-Owned Firms Involved in Hospital
Transactions over a 15-Year Period, 1994–2008**

Acuity Healthcare

Allegiance Health
Management

Alta Healthcare Systems

American Healthcare
Corporation

American Healthcare
Management, Inc.

American Medical
International

American Medical Trust

AmeriHealth

Ardent Health Services

Argilla Healthcare

Attentus Healthcare

Blackstone Group

Blue Cross

Brim Healthcare

Essent Healthcare

FHP International

Fundamental Healthcare

Gillard Healthcare

GP Medical Ventures

Health Management
Associates

Health Mont

Health Plus

HealthTrust

Horizon Health Corporation

Hospital Corporation of
America

IASIS Healthcare

In Med Group

Kohlberg, Kravis, Roberts

Pan American General

Paracelsus

PhyCor

Primary Healthcare

Prime Healthcare

Principal

Province Healthcare

Quorum

Ramsey Health

Renaissance Health Systems

Rural Healthcare
Management

Rx Medical Services

Salick Healthcare

Shelby Medical Holdings

Capella Healthcare

Champion Health

Charter

Cigna

Clarant Hospital Corporation

Columbia

Community Health Systems

Comprehensive Care

Doctors Community Hospital

Dynacq Healthcare

Dynamic Health

Envision Hospital
Corporation

Krug International

Life Point Hospitals

LOCH Holding

Mat Rx Development

Figure 1-2. (Continued)

Medical Professionals of Arizona	Star Health Corporation
	Success Healthcare
Medisphere Health Partners	Summit Health
Merit Health System	Sun Link
National Medical Enterprise	Symphony
Net Care	Tenet
New American Healthcare	Texas Pacific Group
OrNda Hospital Corporation	Transitional Hospital Corporation
Pacer Health Corporation	
Signature Hospital Corporation	Triad
	Universal Health Services
Specialty Hospitals of America	

Source: Modern Healthcare's Annual Report on Mergers and Acquisitions, 1994–2008.

additional companies have also engaged in hospital transitions, but the seventy-eight investor-owned companies listed in this figure have entered into hospital merger or acquisition activity over this period of time. (See Appendix B for a list of those states that have experienced the most merger activity with for-profit companies.)

Mergers form because of financial and market challenges that lead hospital and health system executives and their boards to make decisions that envision a better future in which to fulfill their hospital mission. It is difficult when making such decisions to see very far into the future. It is not unusual for organizations contemplating mergers to "run the numbers" on the expected impact of a merger going out three to five years. Then in making the move to close a merger deal, the anticipated benefits of the merger are touted, usually expressed as cost efficiencies in the form of capital avoidance of duplicative expenditures and improved access to and quality of care, including technology or facility upgrades. If the merger is indeed consummated, hospital executives may announce to their constituents that "nothing will change." One wonders if executives realize that employees and most stakeholders know that hospitals would not merge in the first place if the status quo was to be maintained.

So in the last fifteen years, more than 1,300 community hospital transactions have taken place. Add to this number the big-system regional or national mergers (and the many hospitals that comprise these systems), and one can appreciate how few hospitals and markets have not been affected in some way by merger activity. Given that more than half of these transactions occurred in the mid-1990s, we now have ten to fifteen years of experience on which to look back and examine the impact, outcomes, and lessons learned from health care merger activity.

In this book, we examine both successful and failed mergers, focusing on the reasons, processes, challenges, benefits, and outcomes of these transactions, including the following:

- The drivers in and compelling reasons to pursue a merger
  —How did those reasons bear up with the benefit of hind-sight?
  —Were the reasons, in fact, valid?
- The process to merge: how the transaction was put together
  —Who led the process?
  —Were merger objectives and criteria developed?
  —What outside expertise is required, and when?
  —Was a business plan developed, and when?
  —What does it take to get the deal closed?
- The culture of the organization
  —What is culture?
  —How were cultural issues anticipated and addressed?

—What is leadership's influence and impact on culture?

—How are successful cultures built?

- Naming the new CEO and other leadership considerations

  —What factors affect the question of who will serve as CEO?

  —What considerations must be taken in selection of a new board?

  —What considerations go into selecting the senior management team?

- Outcomes

  —Is the compelling reason to merge always a sound business reason?

  —Do mission, vision, and values really matter?

  —Is it the legal model that makes or breaks a merger?

  —What leadership changes, or retention, occurred in the so-called C-suite?

  —What is the merger's impact on patient care? Did clinical consolidation take place?

The debate about hospital and health care delivery, access, and affordability is again at the forefront of the political agenda. When adding to this discussion the challenges of the U.S. and global economies and the impact that health care cost has on collective competitiveness, the expectation is that merger options will be a necessary strategic discussion for many organizations.

It is our hope and objective that the case studies and stories presented in the following chapters will provide current and future hospital and health system leaders, including trustees, with practical ideas and grounding gleaned from real-world merger experiences to enable their organizations to better prepare to meet their community's health care delivery needs with truly improved access, quality, and competitive cost.

References

1. Sandy Lutz, "Let's Make a Deal," *Modern Healthcare*, 24, no. 51 (December 19, 1994): 47.

2. *Modern Healthcare's Annual Report on Mergers and Acquisitions*, 1994 to 2008. Methodology: Using trends published in *Modern Healthcare's Annual Report on Mergers and Acquisitions*, we eliminated duplicative listings from year to year (e.g., a merger announced one year but closed the following year); we also eliminated deals announced as "pending" but apparently never closed and, where identifiable, eliminated specialty hospitals, such as behavioral health organizations. The focus of our study is the merger activity and experience of acute care hospitals. For purposes of our study and analysis, we defined *transaction* as a merger in which significant changes of control or equity took place, including long-term lease arrangements. Also, relative to not-for-profit versus for-profit entities, any organization that was not investor- (shareholder-) owned we considered to be not-for-profit (e.g., district hospitals would be included in the not-for-profit count).

3. Vince Galloro and Joe Carlson, "Ready for a Resurgence," *Modern Healthcare* (January 18, 2010): 20.

4. David Burda, editor, "By the Numbers," *Modern Healthcare* (December 22, 2008): 72. Thomson Reuters Top 100 Hospitals® was formerly Solucient, an information products company serving the health care industry; Solucient, LLC was acquired by the Thomson Corporation in October 2006. Mease Countryside Hospital is listed as a Top 100 Hospital for 2007 under Large Community Hospitals.

5. Thomson Reuters, "Morton Plant Only U.S. Hospital Awarded Top 100 Honor Every Year, 10 Consecutive Years" [www.mpmhealth.com/blank.cfm?print]. Accessed October 19, 2009.

6. Thomson Reuters, "Heartening Trends," *Modern Healthcare*, 39, no. 46 (November 16, 2009): 32.

7. Using the methodology cited in footnote 2, our compilation indicates that California saw sixty-two mergers in the period from 1994 to 1998. In the period from 1999 to 2008, the state experienced fifty-one mergers, for a fifteen-year total of 113. Texas was a very close second.

8. Thomson Reuters, "Morton Plant," 48, 60.

9. Vince Galloro and Melanie Evans, "HCA Sets New Standard," *Modern Healthcare*, 37, no. 4 (January 22, 2007): 18–19.

10. Dennis K. Berman, "The 100 Largest U.S. Deals of the Decade," *The Wall Street Journal* (December 8, 2009): C1, C3 [http://online. wsj.com/public/resources/documents/st topusdeals 1207 20091206. html]. Accessed December 8, 2009.
11. Ibid.
12. Joe Carlson and Melanie Evans, "No Brakes," *Modern Healthcare* (February 8, 2010): 6.
13. David May, "By the Numbers, 2007–08," *Modern Healthcare* (December 24, 2007): 2.
14. Ibid., 18.

2

Why Merge?

No decision—except the selection of a chief executive officer (CEO)—looms larger for a board than that to merge with another organization. In fact, hiring a CEO is easier than making a decision to merge. Hospitals and health systems do not change their corporate way of conducting business without significant drivers or compelling reasons. The thought of giving up their current state of operation does not come naturally or easily to most organizations. The prospect of losing autonomy, losing board seats, likely restructuring management, and having to anticipate the impact of a merger on employees and the local economy can cause many a sleepless night for CEOs and their boards.

Even when the decision to merge or affiliate appears to be the right choice, by the time this is recognized, some hospitals or health systems have waited too long to make such a move. Sometimes boards convince themselves that time will take care of the present challenge, hoping situations will improve, or perhaps consensus within the board and management to make a change is lacking. Waiting for that hoped-for turnaround often results in an organization trying to negotiate a merger-like transaction from a weakened position. Even worse, some hospitals start down the path toward merger, but before closing the deal, a debate breaks out among the board and with other stakeholders (medical staff and management) as to why they are doing this—a debate that should have taken place and been settled *before* embarking on this path. Many hospitals and some

19

health systems have spent time and money pursuing a merger only to later bring it to a halt because sound reasoning and consensus have been lacking throughout the process.

Equally challenging can be a situation in which strong organizations attempt to determine if a strategic alliance or merger is right for their organization or community. Often a minimal or sometimes even modest "black bottom line" can disguise inherent weaknesses that otherwise calls for a bold move to better position the organization to more effectively compete and provide services in the future. The easy decision is to say "things are going well"; why fix (or change) what is not broken? Standing still is more comfortable and easier—at least for the present.

Though it is management's responsibility to prepare for the board a strategic plan and direction for the organization, it is the board's decision to approve, disapprove, or direct a revision of the plan. The decision to merge, consolidate, or affiliate with another organization is solely one to be made by the board (in the case of faith-based organizations, this final decision may rest with the religious sponsors). It bears repeating that the decision to change the corporate form of doing business is the most important a board will ever make.

To prepare itself for making this decision, the board must understand the environment in which the hospital or health system currently operates and make informed judgments about the current challenges and trends affecting, or potentially affecting, the organization in the context of this environment.

As discussed in chapter 1, more than half of the mergers in the past fifteen years occurred during the five-year period from 1994 to 1998. Let us look at the general characteristics of the health care environment during this time.

The salient aspects of the health care environment of the mid-1990s relating to merger activity were the following:

- Experts throughout the industry believed that *collaboration among health care providers*, rather than competition, would help slow the growth of health care costs. Previous efforts to increase market competition did not seem to slow cost increases, and concerns about them became more pronounced. "You don't need to own it, you just need to influence it" became one working mantra during this period of collaboration. In fact, this author remembers one state hospital association president using the best-selling book *Megatrends 2000,* by John Naisbitt and Patricia Aburdene, as his cornerstone to foster hospital collaboration in his state. One line from that book stands out as an example of the optimism of the pro-collaboration movement: "The post-cold war era will see the United States and the Soviet Union collaborate on the environment and on new nonideological approaches to ending poverty."[1]

- *Managed care* was expected to provide the platform on which price competition would be fostered. With payments made at capitated rates, physicians and hospitals were now responsible for maintaining the health and well-being of a large population base or risk losing money. Hospitals and physicians would compete to win insurance contracts and then have to manage the cost of care within the projected revenue stream of these contracts. This fundamental market belief even led some hospitals and insurance companies to seek mergers with each other. One former hospital ownership company, Humana, converted its business into a managed care plan.

- The *formation of large physician groups* was the fundamental framework by which to attract capital. Physicians and physician groups would have responsibility for patients; they would differentiate themselves by the number and types of specialist, board certification, cost, services, and so on, and they would control the patient experience in the care continuum. Hospitals would seemingly rest at the bottom of the food chain, not much different from one another, as capital and investment would flow to physician groups. In fact, large, publicly traded groups formed and bought many practices, and such firms as PhyCor and Med Partners became familiar names in health care circles. These groups looked to buy not only physician practices but also hospitals. For instance, in 1997, the publicly owned physician practice management company PhyCor bought the Hawaii-based Straub Clinic and Hospital.

- *National health care reform* in the mid-1990s was prominent in the national dialogue. This author had the opportunity to be in the audience when President Bill Clinton kicked off his reform initiative before a live, nationally televised town hall meeting in Tampa, Florida. The initiative eventually would be dubbed "Hillary Care" in response to the leadership by then First Lady Hillary Clinton. Though much of the work of the committee formed to develop the reform package seemed to be conducted in secret, this debate only enhanced the perceived need of hospitals to become part of a bigger entity to compete, creating another factor in the urge to merge.

- *For-profit hospital systems* saw not-for-profit organizations as an opportunity for acquisition or partnership. They also presented another environmental factor for the not-for-profit boards and management to consider—as either an opportunity or a threat. A small firm known as Columbia Healthcare Corporation, whose early years were spent in El Paso, Texas, and parts of Florida, was led by CEO and lawyer Rick Scott, who, during this period, would become the face of for-profit growth activity (discussed in greater depth later in this chapter).

Reasons for Merging

Critical to a hospital or health system management team and board evaluating the strategic merit of a merger or merger-like transaction is to understand the reasons for this consideration—not just general reasons, but very *specific reasons* why *your* organization should consider changing the way it has been conducting its corporate business to date. Each board member should be able to articulate these specific reasons. Usually the CEO is leading this strategic discussion and is in sync with his or her board; however, once again, the decision to merge is the board's alone. Without a strong majority of board members reaching agreement on the compelling reasons to consider merging, embarking down the road to a merger will prove costly and time consuming, with the prospect of failure looming.

The discussion that follows of some common reasons hospitals and health systems consider mergers defines the incentives, or rationale, that lead organizations to come together.

Financial Imperative

In one sense, mergers can be thought of as a legal means to solve a financial problem. Furthermore, one organization's financial problem is often another organization's financial, operational, or market opportunity.

Let us look at how one organization reacted to its environmental assessment. Against the national trends playing out as described, this organization—call it Progressive Health System (an actual case study with the name changed)—owned several medium-sized hospitals. Its flagship was located in an older part of town, while its newest hospital was built in a fast-growing part of the county. Several years of physician dissatisfaction and physician-board tensions within the health system greeted the new CEO upon his arrival. The competitive market was anchored by a larger, financially stronger, well-established not-for-profit entity located just a few miles from Progressive's flagship hospital. Several for-profits had also entered the market, owning or managing hospitals in competition with Progressive. The organization's assessment of its own situation in the context of local, regional, and national trends led it to consider taking on a partner. The form of transaction could be a merger, but the word *partner* sounded better than *merger* to the stakeholders.

The first step taken by the board chair was to form a task force. It was composed of twelve members, including five trustees, four medical staff leaders, one non-trustee community member, the CEO, and one other member of the senior management team. The charge given to the members was "to address the reasons for a partnership/affiliation and to develop the criteria and conditions in order to judge the appropriateness of the partner/affiliation candidates." The board approved hiring a facilitator to assist the group in meeting its charge. Over the next several months, the task force came up with three overarching specific reasons, supported by eighteen points of argument, for Progressive to consider a partnership or an affiliation with another organization. Figure 2-1 sets forth the findings of the task force in answering the "why merge?" question for Progressive Health System.

The board chair then led the task force in a discussion of "partnering," or merging, compared with other alternatives. The choices considered by the group included the following:

1. Not to pursue a partnership or affiliation strategy (go it alone)
2. Put this strategic initiative on hold for a year; see how the operation performs (wait and see strategy)
3. Sell the hospital (likely to a for-profit)
4. Proceed with caution in seeking a strategic partner

The task force felt option 4 made the most sense in the context of its current environment. Thus, the committee completed the first portion of its charge, to articulate the specific reasons (answering the "why merge?" question) to consider a partnership or an affiliation.

The task force presented its findings and recommendations to the board within three months of its formation. Regardless

**Figure 2-1.   Reasons for Progressive Health System's
                Potential Merger**

I.	*High Debt Load*
A	Debt load was high for an organization of its size and revenue base; the organization was challenged to generate enough cash from operations to meet expected capital needs without borrowing.
B	Long-term debt as a percentage of capitalization was 70% versus agency rating of 41%; furthermore, Progressive's long-term debt–to–capitalization ratio was nearly 5 times higher than that of its chief competitor.
C	Annual debt service as a percentage of total revenue was about 8%, compared with the agency rating of 6.7%; its primary competitor's rating was 50% less than that of Progressive.
D	Though the hospital had access to some additional capital, its financial advisers viewed increased borrowing as a high-risk move with little likelihood the incremental debt would be insured.
E	The insurance company, in fact, indicated it would not be interested in insuring new financings.
F	Though outstanding accounts receivable management had generated a decent cash position for Progressive, additional borrowing would be necessary unless operating results came in markedly higher than expected.
II.	*Competitive Position*
A	The entity was not organized effectively to compete for managed care contracts. Physicians began joining the staff of other hospitals to protect their patient and referral base.
B	Though Progressive was one of the lower-cost hospital systems in the region, it did not present enough cost distinction to attract managed care plans on an exclusive provider basis.
C	Employers were accepting less geographic coverage for more cost savings, putting competitors in a better position than that of Progressive.

(Continued on next page)

Figure 2-1.   (Continued)

D	According to two independent consulting reports reviewed by the task force, a competing hospital was the consumer preference in the primary service area.
E	Competitors (for-profit and not-for-profit) were seeking to enter into population growth areas where Progressive currently had facilities and services.
F	A smaller, freestanding not-for-profit hospital was investing heavily in obstetric services, a threat to Progressive's long-standing service at its flagship hospital.
G	A for-profit competitor opened an ambulatory surgery center next to Progressive's newest hospital.
H	Physicians and entrepreneurs would accelerate efforts to take traditional hospital outpatient revenues to alternative settings.
I	The Progressive system lacked critical mass, clinical distinction, and centers of excellence.
III.	**Health Care Environmental Trends**
A	For-profit hospital companies continued to invest within the state.
B	Payers would continue to drive payment incentives to ambulatory settings rather than hospital settings.
C	The American Hospital Association and state hospital associations were encouraging hospitals to collaborate within their communities and regions rather than to compete.
D	Reimbursement systems would likely shift to a fixed-base payment system.

of the outcome, this management and board knew exactly *why* they needed to pursue a different strategic direction. The compelling reasons for this consideration were its high debt load and the risk associated with additional borrowing required to expand its acute care services. With the prospect that hospital consolidation would become more pronounced, positioning itself to access capital would become difficult for the organization without joining a bigger entity.

In summary, financial challenges, especially access to capital, have driven many mergers and acquisitions over the last fifteen years. Progressive Health System was no exception.

Growth Imperative

Organizations need to grow not only to survive but also to thrive and be poised to take advantage of unmet or new market opportunities. Cost cutting is a temporary tactic toward profitability, while cost management is an everyday leadership necessity to navigate the ups and downs of the growth path. Increasing volume and revenue organically, of course, is the ideal approach to market growth, but the fact is, population increases tend to peak at some point, and the ability to gain more customers reaches saturation. Thus, looking at mergers and acquisitions becomes part of an overall strategic consideration to expand markets and/or market share.

We often think of the big organizations as having staying power; however, both large and small systems need to find ways to grow to stay in business, or eventually they risk becoming part of another organization's business. Understanding the implications of the "why merge?" question is equally important in considering growth strategies. An organization might be able to merge its way to growth, but that ability does not necessarily translate to excellence. Two mediocre entities joined together never make one great organization.[2]

Hillcrest Medical Center in Tulsa, Oklahoma, ranked fourth in a four-hospital town in the early 1990s. The CEO, Don Lorack, and his team believed the environmental assessment of that era, which indicated that capitated payments and having to assume responsibility for the health of a large population would indeed become reality. The local environment was such that Hillcrest was the de facto safety net hospital in that region. It was also the only secular, allopathic, not-for-profit hospital in Tulsa. PacifiCare and Blue Cross were the primary insurance providers in the market.[3]

In order to position Hillcrest Medical Center to take responsibility for a large population under the envisioned managed care environment of that era, its leadership needed to find a way to grow, thus establishing its compelling response to the "why merge?" question. In 1994, Hillcrest entered into a full-asset merger with Children's Medical Center of Tulsa and from that platform eventually entered into operating agreements with ten other hospitals in its region.[4]

The for-profit firms have particular appreciation for the need to increase revenues, as the stock market rewards growth, especially profitable growth. Enter Columbia Healthcare Corporation. In the early 1990s, Columbia Healthcare began in El Paso, Texas, and in Florida. Its CEO, Rick Scott, would go on to acquire ninety-five hospitals as the company grew. Columbia's expansion would also maximize profitability in markets where it owned multiple facilities by closing down excess capacity, a strategy that at the time was employed by few other companies, especially not-for-profits.

In 1994, Columbia Healthcare was dubbed "the year's champion of hospital mergers" when it merged its ninety-five hospitals with Hospital Corporation of America's ninety-seven hospitals in a $5.7 million stock swap and changed its name to Columbia/HCA, with Scott continuing as CEO. In the same year, Columbia announced twenty-six individual deals to buy or sell hospitals. To top off the year, newly formed Columbia/HCA announced plans to acquire HealthTrust, another investor-owned company composed of 116 hospitals.[5] In 1995, that deal closed, and by the end of the year, Columbia/HCA had grown to 335 hospitals and 120 ambulatory surgery centers.[6]

The rapid growth of Columbia/HCA and HealthTrust and the expansion activities of other for-profit companies, such as the merger of National Medical Enterprise (NME) with American Medical International (AMI) to form Tenet in 1995, clearly had an impact on the not-for-profit sector. In fact, these mergers were game changers in that they altered the competitive landscape for not-for-profit hospitals, forcing them to create, modify, or intensify their own growth strategies.

Mission Preservation

Finances, or even growth for growth's sake, are not always at the heart of the reason to merge. Sometimes it is in response to a "higher calling." Consider the circumstances and merger drivers that led to the formation of Catholic Health Initiatives (CHI). By the mid-1990s, more than 75 percent of Catholic health care organizations were participating in some type of system structure.[7] However, a wide range of corporate organization models existed among them, characterized by deference to autonomous entities and varying degrees of standardization and centralization of functions.[8] By the early to mid-1990s, a survey conducted by the ten major Catholic systems summarized the competitive imperative: "Contemporary pressures have brought us to a time of change. The need to develop solutions is critical to the vitality of our Catholic health care ministry."[9]

This survey built on earlier work by the Commission on Catholic Health Ministry to seek "significant collaboration with others who share the Church's commitment and new models of sponsorship."[10] In addition, the environmental assessment indicated that for-profit health care was increasingly formidable, and concern was felt within the Catholic health care community that the for-profit sector would take over struggling hospitals.[11]

If vision is the glue that sustains and propels organizations, then vision needs visionaries.

In the formation of CHI, the primary visionaries were Diane Moeller, then CEO of Catholic Health Corporation based in Omaha, Nebraska, and Sister Celestia Koebel, SC, president and CEO of Sisters of Charity Health Care System based in Cincinnati, Ohio.[12] It was at a meeting in mid-1994 with four organizations that were considering coming together that Moeller put the talk of incremental change into a new perspective and vision when she suggested that a giant leap forward should be considered: to consolidate the systems into a large Catholic health care corporation.[13] Moeller and Koebel did not get discouraged when two of the original four organizations dropped out of the discussions. They continued to pursue their vision, believing the merger drivers and reasons to be valid.

They were joined in 1995 by the Franciscan Health System, based in Philadelphia and led by then CEO Ron Aldrich. Though each CEO was running a successful system, each took the risk and believed the signs of the times called for a new structure to preserve the ministry of Catholic health care. As Aldrich is quoted as saying, "Originally the idea of CHI belonged to the three CEOs [Moeller, Koebel, and Aldrich]. However, the religious congregations embraced it so enthusiastically that they soon took the lead, then thereafter the CEOs followed."[14]

Such mission preservation and continuation is embraced by organizations beyond those with faith-based structures. Chief Executive Officer Pat Fry of Sutter Health, a not-for-profit, secular Sacramento-based system of twenty-four hospitals in northern California, describes the pivotal event in what he calls the "Phase I" days when the Sacramento hospitals were known as Sutter Community Hospitals. In those days, after turning around two hospitals, merging assets, and reconfiguring the board, the board outlined its fundamental principle that not-for-profit health care needed to be protected and fostered.[15]

This philosophy emerged at a time when for-profit interest was both evident and rumored in the Sacramento-area market. However, the Sutter board decided that no check a for-profit company could write was big enough to relinquish its ideal of protecting not-for-profit health care.[16]

In somewhat similar fashion, the formation of the BayCare Health System in Florida was spawned by the "desire to preserve community-owned health care availability" in the wake of encroaching for-profit-owned and -managed facilities in the Tampa Bay region.[17] The establishment of BayCare through a joint operating agreement in 1996 included nine community hospitals, two of which are Catholic hospitals and one of which is a Baptist hospital. The compelling reason to merge—preserving community-owned health care—became the source that continues to sustain BayCare's success to this day.

Defensive Position

Sometimes mergers are contemplated and entered into for defensive reasons. They can take on several forms and become the answer to "why merge?"

Bernie Brown, former CEO of PROMINA Health System in Atlanta, believes "Mergers occur for one of two reasons. Leaders either like each other or they have a common enemy."[18] In the case of PROMINA in the mid-1990s, that enemy was a joint venture between Emory University's health care system and HCA. The fear it generated compelled other organizations to consider becoming part of a bigger entity to compete.[19]

Another community hospital CEO refers to the impact of "lunatics" in the market. The term in this case refers to the Allegheny Health, Education and Research Foundation (AHERF), the Pittsburgh-based organization that aggressively reached beyond the city to buy hospitals and physician practices in the Philadelphia area. This activity led the above-mentioned CEO's medical staff to fear that the physicians from the "big city" would soon be coming to take their suburban jobs.

The CEO's experience in this climate led him to believe that the presence of a lunatic organization in the marketplace causes "the rest of the world to react." In response, his hospital merged with a different organization, a large teaching hospital three counties away from Philadelphia, a move considered to be a good defensive strategy to put distance between it and the big-city hospitals and physicians. The large teaching hospital also saw the merger as a defensive move, to protect its

eastern market area. Less than five years into the merger, however, both parties agreed it was a failure. Moreover, the aggressive organization known as AHERF ended up in a colossal
bankruptcy, a well-documented case study unto itself.

Defensive mergers can be fraught with challenges. Such
mergers often lack an offensive plan—one that commits to
investment and growth—leaving the organizations vulnerable
to failure. Larger organizations sometimes enter into defensive
mergers to preclude another organization from merging or buying smaller facilities, with no real intent on developing services.
For the smaller organization, defensive mergers often translate
into slow death if a strategic growth plan is not put in place.

One CEO described his negotiations with a larger organization. Though some aspects of the proposed business combination presented an attractive strategic partner, other aspects of
the deal appeared to pit the two organizations against each
other in a number of areas. Frustrated at being unable to
gain clarity on the situation, the CEO of the smaller facility
succinctly put his merger objective on the table to the other
organization when he stated, "You can be my partner, or you
can be my competitor, but you can't be both. You choose." The
discussions ended shortly thereafter.[20]

Sometimes the defensive cause that drives the "why" of a
merger is a reaction to legal or regulatory pressures. Such, at
least in part, was the case with the National Medical Enterprise merger with American Medical International mentioned
earlier. The trouble for NME began in 1991 when the Texas
attorney general sued the organization for allegedly overbilling
at its psychiatric facilities. Patients and insurance companies
filed suits accusing NME of insurance fraud. In August 1993,
Federal Bureau of Investigation agents raided NME's head-
quarters and several of its psychiatric facilities. By 1994, after
spending considerable time and money in legal proceedings,
the company reached a settlement with the government and
sold off most of its psychiatric facilities to refocus on the acute

care business. The merger with AMI in 1995 allowed NME to reincarnate itself into Tenet Healthcare Corporation, a name meant to reflect the combined company's rigorously principled approach to business.[21]

The 1999 merger of Alta Bates (part of Sutter) with Summit Medical Center located in Oakland, California, was, according to CEO Warren Kirk, at least in part defensive.[22] The two organizations had competed vigorously for patients and physicians. Kirk became CEO of Alta Bates in the middle of the discussions with Summit and recalls that Summit was allegedly also in discussions with a for-profit entity. The two organizations did, in fact, merge after an antitrust challenge and remain a successful entity.

Merge (or Sell) Rather than Close

Missions are not forever. Advances in medical science may reduce or eliminate the need for particular services or treatments. For example, at one time, some hospitals operated solely for the treatment of tuberculosis. These hospitals were eventually closed or converted as the medical need for this focused specialty was no longer warranted given the advances in treatment and prevention. The March of Dimes originally focused its charity efforts on polio; when this disease was virtually eliminated, the organization changed its mission to "[improving] the health of babies by preventing birth defects, premature birth, and infant mortality."[23]

But most hospital managers and boards have difficulty coming to grips with a declining need for hospital services. Mention the possibility of a hospital closing, and chances are, the politicians, eyeing votes, along with community groups will have a renewed interest in keeping it open. Numerous acute care hospitals have seen better opportunities to merge in earlier times, but given their desire to hold onto their autonomy, a continuing market decline later leaves them with little leverage in seeking a merger partner. When these hospitals merge, they tend to undergo what looks more like an acquisition than a true merger, basically a going-out-of-business sale.

One of the more prudent decisions made while contemplating merging, closing, or another use of management and capital investment was made by CEO Kevin Leahy and the board at the Sisters of St. Francis Health System in Mishawaka, Indiana, in 1997. Having asked a turnaround firm to review his operations at St. Joseph Hospital in Memphis, Tennessee, Leahy and the board came to realize that a sustainable operation would involve a substantial commitment of time and money into the only hospital the system owned in the state. After quickly reviewing and deliberating on the report findings, the board and CEO reached a difficult and emotional decision to try to sell St. Joseph Hospital. The emotional choice was compounded by the sisters' deep and lengthy connection to the ministry in Memphis and concern for the employees.

Furthermore, this hospital had historical relevance, as it was where the Reverend Martin Luther King Jr. was taken when he was shot in 1968, fulfilling his wish, according to stories reported to Leahy, that if he were ever injured he wanted to be treated at a Catholic hospital.[24]

Nevertheless, the difficult decision was made to sell, and as the former outside attorney, John Swartz, recalls, Leahy called him on October 1, 1997, to share the news. When Swartz asked who the prospective buyers were, Leahy reported, "None."[25]

A short time later, Leahy recalled walking toward the CEO suite at St. Jude Hospital to meet with that organization's CEO and on his way noticed a model of planned expansion for St. Jude. The expansion had been delayed because the St. Jude property was locked in between St. Joseph Hospital and a highway. He recalls thinking to himself he had a chance when he saw the expansion plans. Indeed, St. Jude was interested in a deal, but only for the land and buildings. Leahy then went to Baptist Health System, whose downtown hospital had plenty of capacity and found that, indeed, it was interested in St. Joseph's hospital business. Leahy subsequently closed a three-way deal: St. Jude bought the land and buildings, and Baptist bought the hospital business. Most of the St. Joseph employees were retained. The sisters left a different mission behind in Memphis, working with Baptist on faith-based initiatives in such areas as nursing scholarships and housing for AIDS patients.

The three-way transaction was orchestrated in a timely fashion, with the deal completed within sixty days, on November 30, 1997. It proved to be a winning strategy for all three parties and an unusually positive outcome to the "merge or sell rather than close" scenario.[26] Sometimes the mission is simply over, and it is best to recognize this fact and conclude it or change it.

In summary, the reason for merging often transcends the above categories, but typically one of these five reasons— financial imperative, growth imperative, mission preservation, defensive position, or merge/sell rather than close—becomes the predominant driver answering the question "why merge?"

Trends or Fads: Both Are Factors in the "Why Merge?" Scenario

Discerning between a trend and a fad is difficult in the short run. Sports enthusiasts know that certain professional sports are known as "copy cats" because they adopt strategies and tactics from successful teams. The same is true in health care, where the latest news from the Web sites of consulting or advisory firms and the front pages of hospital professional journals may spur a reaction from executives of health systems, hospitals, and physician practices. For instance, a generation ago, "corporate reorganization" became a must-follow activity or fad, with many hospitals forming different corporate entities. The ultimate value of these activities was questionable in many circumstances. The same movement was seen in the 1990s with the rush to adopt hospital operational "reengineering" projects, whereby the clients were many for various consulting firms. Similarly, the sustainable value of these efforts was often found wanting.

Let us review what really happened in the dynamic national health care environment that dominated the 1990s and led to the largest number of hospital mergers ever experienced up to that time or since. Again, more than half of the mergers that have taken place in the last fifteen years occurred in the five-year period between 1994 and 1998.

Managed Care

Clearly the fear—or perhaps the opportunity—of capitation payments being made to large physician groups and hospitals caused health care executives to consider how they would manage the health of a large population base inside of a defined revenue stream. This reaction resulted in hospitals implementing a number of strategies or tactics, as discussed below.

The purchase of physician practices became an "own it or lose it" competition. Physicians, who never dreamed of becoming employees, were now salaried by hospitals or other entities, such as publicly traded physician practice management firms.

In addition, some hospitals either started managed care plans or joined with others in forming managed care plans. In essence, hospitals were now in the insurance business.

Finally, hospitals merged with other hospitals to position themselves to take care of a larger population base and to survive in the impending capitated environment. What was the outcome? Was this a trend or a fad?

The capitation "monster" did not develop as anticipated or feared. The public's negative reaction to health maintenance organization (HMO) steering compromised the anticipated spread of West Coast–style capitation; thus, it simply did not materialize to the extent articulated by futurists or consultants.

In addition, the purchase of physician practices by hospitals proved costly, as hospital executives learned through difficult experience that running physician practices, with their smaller unit and dollar volumes, is different from running a hospital. Many hospitals lost significant amounts of money as a result of buying and managing these practices, so much so that the threshold of success became defined by a hospital losing only $100,000 per physician. Furthermore, the publicly traded physician practice management companies, PhyCor and Med Partners, went out of business. The Straub Clinic and Hospital in Hawaii, mentioned in chapter 1, bought back its assets from PhyCor in 2000, the merger deal having lasted only three years.[27]

If these lessons were not costly enough, getting into the insurance business proved to be an even more costly education. The metric for success was market share, but many failed to recognize that, absent tight cost management, increasing market share with an increasingly higher cost structure was a failed strategy. One does not make up such losses on volume, and it was volume that was prized.

Of course, not all activity was a fad. In many cases hospitals that merged were able to pool their financial strength and intellectual capital to improve their negotiating position with large, well-financed insurance companies. Notwithstanding this important aspect, clearly the "bogeyman" of managed care capitation and the strategies and tactics undertaken to deal with what was seen as an inevitable environment simply proved not to be the disruption that was predicted. Furthermore, hospitals, once thought to be a commodity, were in fact the financial engine holding up the rest of the corporate organizations (physician practices, insurance companies, home health agencies, real estate corporations, and so on) formed to respond to the market dynamics of the day.

For-Profit Hospital Growth

Possibly no dynamic caused not-for-profits to think more about mergers or affiliation than the environmental factor of for-profit hospital growth. Hospital CEOs and their boards considered either merging with a for-profit company or joining up with other not-for-profits. For-profit alternatives were seen as either an opportunity or a threat. As indicated earlier, Columbia/HCA and other for-profit hospital systems often became the compelling reason to enter into these discussions. One for-profit executive challenged faith-based organizations not to put all their eggs in one (hospital) basket. The argument went that a number of religious sponsors had not begun their enterprises in the hospital business, so their ministry might best be protected by taking less of an interest in hospitals or shifting priorities to other areas of need.[28]

Some boards made the decision to leave the not-for-profit hospital business, as it was fraught with the challenges of managing medical staff relationships and executive turnover. Often the sale of the hospital created a community foundation to use for other charitable health care initiatives.

As to the for-profit companies, Wall Street rewards increasing revenues and profitability, and without organic growth, the for-profit companies needed to look to alternative strategies, including merging with other systems. The outcome of this intense pressure and the related publicity of several government investigations caused trouble for some firms such as Tenet and Columbia/HCA. Today, the for-profit sector comprises less than 20 percent of the total nonfederal, short-term acute care hospitals in the United States.

The for-profit takeover fad did seem to bring a more pronounced business focus to the not-for-profit sector. On the one hand, a fair number of not-for-profits pulled together to form affiliations and mergers to protect the value and contribution of not-for-profit health care. On the other hand, they saw the for-profit companies taking over ailing not-for-profit hospitals and making them profitable. For-profits brought a certain discipline, standardization, and accountability to achieving results. However, overall, the phenomenon of for-profit hospital expansion and encroachment was not nearly as pronounced as was feared by not-for-profits.

"Hillary Care"

The need for national health care reform was a key component of President Clinton's national agenda in the mid-1990s. His appointment of the first lady to head up the planning for this reform and the activities her committee embarked on led to significant publicity. This reform initiative and the existing managed care environment, combined with the for-profit sector activity, only served to further fuel consideration of mergers. With the focus on how to insure the 40 million people without coverage, and with HMO "gatekeepers" already souring many Americans on this process of accessing care, health care reform failed to make a compelling case as to how government-led initiatives with hard-to-understand matrixes could make an already complex system appreciably better for the majority of Americans who already enjoyed some sort of insurance coverage. As a result, the Clinton health care reform package did not move forward.

The Board's Role in Critiquing the "Why Merge?" Consideration

So how are a management team and board to interpret the national and local industry trends and make a decision to either stay the course or change direction and consider a merger-like transaction? After all, health care is considered by many to be local rather than national in scope.

The challenge for the board is to view the industry long term. Management teams tend to develop strategic plans encompassing a relatively short time frame of three to five years. Furthermore, compensation is usually based on similarly short-term objectives. Boards, on the other hand, bring the depth and breadth of various industry trends and life cycles and continuity of community involvement to the boardroom that should enable them to ask the questions that assist management in reaching sound conclusions about the direction of a hospital or health system. Board members must communicate their experiences in the boardroom, ask questions, and make decisions. This is their fiduciary duty.

In deliberating the merits and reality of a strategic plan and, indeed, making judgments as to how national trends or fads might affect a local market, it is wise for a board to ask certain types of questions related to its strategic plan, as listed in figure 2-2.

The board and management must take its local situation and evaluate its future through the filter of regional and national trends affecting the health care delivery system. Leaders must assess the national health care environment factors for trends versus fads (figure 2-3).

Figure 2-2.   Questions for Monitoring the Strategic Plan's Progress

1	What are the organization's critical success factors (measurable milestones)?
2	Are we on target with agreed-upon strategic milestones?
3	Does the annual budget significantly correlate to the strategic plan? Do the investments called for in the strategic plan make it to the budget and actually occur?
4	Does the actual operating and financial performance meet or exceed budget?
5	If the organization is underperforming, why? Is the strategic plan credible?
6	If the organization is exceeding performance, how can we accelerate clinical competence and competitive position? How does the organization prevent itself from becoming too comfortable with its success, thus missing opportunities?
7	What specific local or regional factors are enhancing or impeding the organization's performance, such as physician recruitment and retention; clinical reputation; patient satisfaction; medical staff relationships; nursing recruitment and turnover; employee retention; local economy; changing market, employer, and insurance dynamics; management stability; or other strengths and weaknesses?

Do the answers to the questions in figure 2-3 (or other similar questions) call for staying the course or for evaluating alternative strategies? The outcome should be for the board to consider an objective assessment—a report card—of its organization (figure 2-4).

In which direction is your organization heading? Perhaps the results of the exercises demonstrated in figures 2-3 and 2-4 and earlier discussions will lead a health system or hospital to realize it needs to seriously consider going in a different direction.

Figure 2-3. Questions for Distinguishing Trends versus Fads

1	Have these factors or trends appeared before? If so, what happened?
2	If these factors are essentially correct, what is the impact on our system or hospital?
3	If these factors are only half correct, which half are most likely to be correct, and what is the impact on our system or hospital?
4	If these national factors are essentially fads and not trends, what, if any, affect results?

Figure 2-4. Strategic Plan Report Card Questions

1	Are we on target and meeting critical success factors and milestones?
2	Does the actual operating and financial performance meet/exceed budget?
3	What specific local or regional factors are *enhancing* performance?
4	What specific local or regional factors are *impeding* performance?
5	Do we size up the health care competitive environment as trends versus fads?
6	Are we a growing business, a stable business, or slowly going out of business?

If the organization is able to come out of such a deliberation understanding why a merger or merger-like transaction must be considered, then a critical first step to a successful transition will have been accomplished.

References

1. John Naisbitt and Patricia Aburdene, *Megatrends 2000* (New York: William Morrow, 1990), 313.
2. Jim Collins, *Good to Great: Why Some Companies Make the Leap . . . and Others Don't* (New York: HarperCollins, 2001), 181.
3. Don Lorack, former CEO, Hillcrest Health System, interview with author, Orange County, California, July 17, 2009.
4. Ibid.
5. Sandy Lutz, "Let's Make a Deal," *Modern Healthcare* (December 19, 1994): 47.
6. Sandy Lutz, "1995: A Record Year for Hospital Deals," *Modern Healthcare* (December 18, 1995): 44.
7. Patricia A. Cahill and Maryanna Coyle, *Catholic Health Initiatives, a Spirit of Innovation, a Legacy of Care, the Early Years* (Denver: Catholic Health Initiatives, 2006), 2.
8. Ibid., 22.
9. Ibid., 3.
10. Ibid., 3.
11. Ibid., 22.
12. Ibid., 23.
13. Ibid., 24.
14. Ibid., 30–31.
15. Patrick Fry, CEO, Sutter Health, interview with author, Sacramento, California, July 20, 2009.
16. Scott McMurray, *Building a System, the History of Sutter Health* (Sacramento, CA: Sutter Health, 2006), 45.
17. Phillip K. Beauchamp, former CEO, Mease Healthcare, and former CEO, Morton Plant Mease Health, interview with author, Dunedin, Florida, June 26, 2009.
18. Bernard L. (Bernie) Brown, telephone interview with author, July 7, 2009.
19. Bernard L. (Bernie) Brown, interview with author, Atlanta, July 16, 2009.
20. James Thornton, former CEO, Brandywine Hospital, interview with author, Media, Pennsylvania, July 21, 2009.
21. Answers.com, "Hoover's Profile: Tenet Healthcare Corporation" [http://www.answers.com/topic/tenet-healthcare-corporation]. Accessed July 3, 2009.

22. Warren Kirk, CEO, Alta Bates Summit, interview with author, Oakland, California, July 22, 2009.
23. March of Dimes, "About Us" [http://www.marchofdimes.com/787 .asp]. Accessed February 22, 2010.
24. Kevin Leahy, CEO, Sisters of St. Francis Health System, interview with author, August 17, 2009.
25. John Swartz, attorney, Sisters of St. Francis Health System, interview with author, August 17, 2009.
26. Leahy interview.
27. Deanna Bellandi, "The Deals Are Off," *Modern Healthcare* (January 8, 2001): 44.
28. David T. Vandewater, president and CEO, Ardent Health Services, interview with author, August 27, 2009.

3

What Do We Want from a Merger—and How Do We Get There?

Once a health system or hospital determines that its strategic direction calls for consideration of a merger with another health system or hospital, the next important deliberation is to ascertain specifically what it expects a merger to accomplish. In short, *what are the objectives of the merger?*

Unrealistic expectations, ill-considered or poorly prepared objectives, or a compromised process can derail a transaction, thus setting back the desired strategic objectives of the organization. For example, let us review some mergers announced over the years:

- Mercy Hospital in Miami and the then four-hospital system Baptist Health South Florida sign a letter of intent to merge in 1996.[1] The deal never occurs, and three years later Mercy becomes part of Catholic Health East.[2]

- Newnan Hospital (253 beds) and Peachtree Regional Hospital (144 beds), the only two hospitals in Newnan, Georgia, agree to merge in 1995.[3] The move seems to make sense to observers. But instead of merging, one year later, Newnan Hospital signs a letter of intent to form a 50-50 joint venture with for-profit Columbia.[4] However, it is Peachtree Regional that ends up in a joint venture with Columbia and Emory University Hospital. The

story becomes more interesting when in 2002 Newnan
Hospital acquires Peachtree Regional from HCA and
Emory.[5] The saga continues when in 2007 Newnan is
bought by Piedmont Medical Center in Atlanta.[6]

- In 1995, Columbia enters into a joint venture with the
Sisters of Charity of St. Augustine Health System in
Cleveland. The deal includes hospitals in Ohio and South
Carolina.[7] Are the objectives and cultures compatible
between the national for-profit and the regional faith-
based Catholic system? Some four years later, the University Hospitals Health System in Cleveland steps in and
replaces Columbia as the 50 percent joint venture partner
for the Ohio hospitals.[8]

- In New Orleans in 1994, Mercy and Southern Baptist
hospitals merge to become the largest private hospital in
the city.[9] One year later, the for-profit company Tenet
buys Mercy-Baptist for $222 million.[10]

- In 1997, in Nashville, Tennessee, St. Thomas Health Services (514 beds) and Baptist Hospital (649 beds) agree "to
create an integrated parent company in a deal expected
to be completed early this year."[11] The deal does close—
four years later, with St. Thomas acquiring Baptist in an
asset purchase.[12]

- In West Palm Beach, Florida, in 2000 the board of trustees of a two-hospital system, Intracoastal, approves an
agreement to change the management and governance in
order for Catholic Health East to become the sole owner.
The deal is expected to be completed by March 15,
2002.[13] However, in 2001, the not-for-profit Intracoastal
sells its two hospitals to for-profit Tenet.[14]

- In the state of Washington, Swedish Medical Center in
Seattle announces a definitive agreement to merge in
1994 with Tacoma-based MultiCare Health System.[15]
The deal never closes.

Merger Objectives

A good place for a health system or hospital to start in contemplating realistic merger objectives is to determine what advantages it has to offer a prospective partner and—equally important— to be candid about the impediments (baggage) it also brings to the deal table. Sometimes a facilitator, or third party, is helpful in assisting a board and management team to objectively assess the organization's strengths and weaknesses in the context of a potential transaction. Figure 3-1 shows how Progressive Health System (a real case with the name of the organization changed; introduced in chapter 2) sized up its situation.

Having previously agreed on reasons for considering a merger and examined both the advantages and potential burdens the organization might bring to a deal, its leadership articulated the overarching objectives it sought in a merger transaction (figure 3-2).

One may argue the merits of the advantages and disadvantages defined by this small health system in the heyday of merger mania in the mid-1990s, but the point is that this is an organization that knew why it needed to merge and what it wanted out of a merger. If it were to determine a merger would not meet its objectives, the organization was prepared to walk away and look at other alternatives.

Merger Criteria: What Kind of Organization Fits the Merger Objectives?

Once an organization knows why it wants to merge and what it seeks from a merger (merger objectives), the next key step is to develop criteria by which to judge prospective merger partners. Developing criteria early on saves time, energy, and money in a process that can quickly become more emotional than rational. It allows an organization to focus on *what* is important and *who* (which organizations) might serve the organization's strategic purpose. Equally important, early criteria development provides

Figure 3-1. Progressive Health System's Strength/Weakness Assessment Process

Advantages Progressive Health System has to offer a potential partner
- An undersized hospital in a growing, attractive community, part of underserved service area
- Both significant and improving market share in its newest campus location
- Profitable hospital operations; recent improvement in utilization and financial performance
- Sound base of respected admitting physicians, board certified and covering most medical and surgical subspecialties
- Good reputation among physicians, consumers, and insurance plans
- Good physician relations
- Board of trustees' desire to do what is best for community in providing health services to primary markets served by the system
- Improving relations between board and medical staff
- Good management team

Disadvantages or impediments Progressive Health System presents to a potential partner
- Mature population in several markets
- Small health system lacking in geographic breadth
- Large amount of debt, combined with significant need for capital
- Several well-capitalized not-for-profit and for-profit competitors
- Debt covenants that compromise organizational and corporate flexibility
- Potential erosion of medical staff joining staff of other hospitals, especially primary competitor
- Weak managed care infrastructure on part of both hospital and physicians
- Significant vacant space in its flagship medical office building
- Aging facility at flagship location
- Potential antitrust issues, depending on partner selected

Figure 3-2. Objectives of a Partnership Strategy for Progressive Health System

- Ensure the long-term strength and success of Progressive to meet its mission of delivering health care services to its primary service area
- Gain access to capital, particularly to expand its newest campus
- Achieve operating and capital savings through shared technology, shared purchasing, and consolidation of services where practical
- Improve attractiveness for managed care contracting, including physician organization and primary care recruitment
- Improve clinical capability and coordination of service delivery, focusing on patient and physician needs and convenience
- Improve image of Progressive through a merger or an affiliation that will provide top-of-mind awareness and clinical distinction in the market
- Preserve local autonomy, governance, and management to the extent possible, consistent with the partnership strategy
- Local board and management participation in overall system strategic planning and decision making

an organization with a rational framework by which to decide to walk away from suitor organizations that do not meet its objectives and criteria. Having a rational approach based on using well-developed criteria is important in a process that can become subjective in a negotiating room full of executive egos.

One chief executive officer (CEO) who concluded, with the support of the board, that the hospital needed to find a merger partner used what he called his "four Cs" for consolidation or merger criteria (figure 3-3).[16]

Our case study health system, Progressive, developed its criteria around seven themes, believing these to correlate with its answers to the question "why merge?" (see chapter 2) and with the objectives it sought from a merger partner, as outlined in figure 3-4. Effective leaders link merger criteria back to their compelling reasons ("why merge?") and merger objectives.

Figure 3-3.   Four Cs for Consolidation or Merger

Capability	Clinical strength, culture
Capital	Financial strength, access to capital dollars
Clout	Negotiating clout, position of strength in dealing with health plans
Computers	Technology advances, functionality

The substance or detail of Progressive's criteria may be subject to debate, but by setting out the criteria, Progressive signals that any potential strategic partner would be dealing with a hospital organization that has deliberated sufficiently on its current and likely future state and knows the outcome it wants to achieve from a merger. This is a prepared organization, and such preparation usually serves an organization very well. In fact, organizations like Progressive may have to wait for interested and even bigger organizations, which often consider themselves sophisticated at such transactions, to catch up. As a former colleague of the author and many sports observers have said, Hockey Hall of Fame great Wayne Gretzky never skated to where the puck was; he skated to where the puck was going—a key to his success.

A prepared health system or hospital knows the strategic road to take and the forks in the road to be avoided. It is heading to the future with confidence. Figure 3-5 summarizes some key decision points to address when preparing for a merger.

How to Get the Deal Done

As large as the health care industry is, many who work in it consider it small, especially in the hospital sector. This is because it is characterized by its relationships. It is about personal reputation, integrity, and passion for mission and service, regardless of profit status.

Figure 3-4. Screening Criteria for Selecting a Strategic Partner for Progressive Health System

I	Geographic Preference (in order of preference)
	Local
	National
II	Type of Organization (in order of preference)
	Not-for-profit secular
	Religious affiliation (not-for-profit)
	Investor-owned organization
III	Size of Strategic Partner
	Minimum of 500 beds (stand alone or system)
	Occupancy: average above 70% last 5 years
	Breadth of services: tertiary clinical capabilities
	System experience demonstrated via: • Number of hospitals in current system • Number of years operating as a system
	If system is inexperienced, lacks sufficient track record: • Negotiate greater board representation • Consider trial period of affiliation before proceeding further
IV	Physician Development/Teaching Programs (if partner has teaching programs)
	Focus on primary care development (regardless of teaching affiliation or absence of affiliation)
	Participation of Progressive Health System hospitals as site for intern/resident training with preferred emphasis on family practice
	Participation of Progressive physicians in teaching programs
V	Managed Care
	Track record of successful managed care experience (number of contracts, lives covered, and number of primary and specialist participants)
	Track record of efficient and effective utilization and case management
	Demonstrated ability to manage care (outcomes) on a profitable basis
	Demonstrated community commitment to prevention and wellness programs
	Appropriate commitment to meeting indigent care needs, demonstrated charity care experience rendered over last 5 years

(Continued on next page)

Figure 3-4.   (Continued)

VI	**Profitability of Target Health System or Hospital**
	Dominant market share in its primary service area and significant market share in secondary service areas
	Track record of good historical financial performance: minimum of 3% operating margin over last 5 years
	Debt-to-equity ratio: less than 45%
	Capital expense ratio: less than 9%
	Admitting patterns stable or growing over last 5 years
	Outpatient revenue: growth in business over last 5 years, with demonstrated innovation in ambulatory care placement and development
	Demonstrated appropriate level of investments in technology and physical plant over last 5 years, combined with sound financing strategy
	Compliance with all bond or loan covenants
	Cash position: minimum of 100 days, cushion ratio of 2.5:1, and accounts receivable turnover (days outstanding) less than 70
	Agency rating of A or better
	Prospects for future financial viability are sound, considering historical performance, existing certificate-of-need applications, and projected financial/operational performance
VII	**Corporate Culture of Target Strategic Partner**
	Team orientation organization with demonstrated history of collegial relationships combined with appropriate and timely decision-making process among board, medical staff, and management
	Demonstrated commitment to mission of community hospitals
	Decentralized style of management evidenced by: • Low corporate overhead • Management fee/overhead allocation formula known ahead of time, understood, and reviewed for appropriateness on an annual basis
	Commitment to a continuous quality improvement program
	Ability to resolve sensitive issues affecting medical staff, such as credentialing, recruitment, and hospital-based physician contracts

Figure 3-5. Merger Preparation for Management and Board

Why merge?	List specific drivers/compelling reasons.
Advantages	Ask, What do we bring to the table?
Impediments	Flesh out issues/baggage that may compromise the other's interest.
Merger objectives	Identify what is needed out of a merger/ what must be gained.
Screening criteria	Determine how to judge the appropriateness of prospective partners.

In most cases, prospecting for a strategic partner rests with the CEO, who is tasked by the board to carry out the organization's strategic and operational directives and to protect the mission, purpose, and assets of the organization. The board confers final approval on such actions, but the CEO and his or her team carry out the day-to-day responsibilities.

Importantly, as we have seen in this and previous chapters, preparation and teamwork usually make a better case for success. One CEO of a four-hospital system located in the Mid-Atlantic region is, at the time of this writing, negotiating a merger with another system. He set out on his own and found what he believed to be the ideal merger partner and then reported back to the board. This report was the first mention the board had encountered of a merger. The merger may work—or it may not. Earlier in the 2000s, a CEO of a system in the South was running an organization of a half dozen hospitals built through mergers and acquisitions that eventually fell into financial trouble. He sought a deal to sell to a for-profit company and believed, with the backing of the executive committee, he had found the ideal strategic buyer. However, when the details of this proposed transaction were presented to the entire board, its surprise and dismay to learn of this deal led to the CEO's dismissal. The lesson here is for a CEO to avoid getting out too far in front of the organization's board. It is important that both the "why merge?"

and the "who do we merge with?" questions be considered with the board's participation and concurrence.

On the other hand, it is rarely a good practice for a board to negotiate a merger independent of its CEO and key senior leaders. One executive, experienced in several mergers (some well managed, some not) related this story: The management team, including the CEO, was informed by the board leadership on a Friday afternoon of a merger deal being closed the following Monday morning. It was the first the management team, including the CEO; employees; and medical staff had learned of the decision. Shock was the only word the CEO had to describe the experience. The hospital had been through a successful turnaround and the feeling of employees was one of overwhelming betrayal. Amazingly, in a transaction conducted in secret by the board, the management team was kept on following the merger. It spent the entire first year in the merged entity dealing with employee shock, anger, and grief. Now three years into the merger, the medical staff still harbor deep resentment about the merger and the process that was used to reach the decision for the hospital to merge. Such a decision certainly rests with the board in the end, but a steep price has been paid for the communication tactics chosen in excluding its management team and medical leadership in the process.

Facilitator: Is One Needed?

Usually, with the board's blessing, the CEO makes initial contact with prospective strategic partners. Most merger transactions are, in fact, CEO driven. Sometimes, however, a facilitator may be hired to work with the organization(s). This individual could be a financial adviser, a consultant, a lawyer—someone seen as having the objectivity, professional experience, and reputation to represent one or more parties. The facilitator will work with both parties, and any additional entities if multiple potential partners are considering merger or consolidation.

As indicated in the discussion in chapter 2 of the formation of Catholic Health Initiatives, hiring a capable and respected attorney as facilitator was considered "the wisest and most valuable decision" the organization made in the process. In the merger process, the facilitator was able to "navigate the agenda and group dynamics with ease, knowing when to let the energy flow and when to re-channel it into reality."[17]

An organization that considers using the services of a facilitator must be discerning in its choice of adviser. Be sure third parties are not impeding a process in which management and board (and perhaps sponsors) need to be talking *with* each other directly, and not *through* a facilitator. There comes a time when a facilitator needs to drop back and allow the organization's leadership to have the difficult conversations that take place in any merger transaction. Potential merger partners must spend sufficient time early in the process to get to know each other (while respecting antitrust guidelines, discussed later in the chapter), which will help the deal move from discussion to finalization and closure.

A good facilitator is also mindful of motives and hidden agendas. A facilitator works closely with the CEO and the leadership team appointed to oversee the selection or to bring together with the organization a strategic merger partner (see the next section). Sometimes a party agrees to a facilitator because it has been caught up in a merger discussion and frankly does not want to merge but does not know how to say no (and likely wants to keep the door open for the future). It is this party's hope that the facilitator will determine the merger does not make sense. A skilled facilitator recognizes situations in which one or more parties are not revealing their true motivation and agendas. In such cases, the negotiation process should end.

Merger Negotiating Committee

Often a leadership group is appointed and approved by the board (or sponsors) to screen potential merger candidates and to enter into detailed discussions with the final one or two organizations in contention as a merger partner. This group is often called a task force or steering committee and consists of the CEO, the chief financial officer, board leadership, key medical staff leadership, and sponsors for religious organizations. This group will make the merger recommendation to the board. For-profit companies usually form smaller task forces or committees for this purpose, as many have significant merger experience. The same is not true of most not-for-profits, and thus the importance of the strategic merger decision tends to lend itself to more participants at the table.

Great care needs to be taken in the selection of the leadership that comprises the merger committee. Sometimes the team selected is the executive committee of the organization; in other cases it is the task force that determined the merger objectives and was involved in fulfilling the earlier charge to answer "why merge?" Some bigger systems have transaction or transition committees that evaluate merger or partner opportunities.

Regardless, it is critical to get the right people with the right skills to serve on the merger negotiating committee. One CEO conveyed this story: A merger negotiation proceeded successfully only to have a key physician who sat through the process glean all of the strategic information and then enlist a group of doctors to build a hospital to compete with the newly merged entity. Other mergers have been derailed by longtime board members who, when realizing a merger discussion was gaining traction and not wanting it to happen, placed calls to the press or took other untoward action. Be certain that the right people with skill, judgment, objectivity, and integrity are involved and that they understand merger decisions are often the biggest decisions in the life of a management team and board—if not on your side of the negotiating table, then likely on the other side.

Sensitivity is a requirement. "Winning" at the negotiating table is one thing, but the key objective is to make the transaction actually work when the deal is closed.

Cost of a Merger

An old carpenter saying cautions, "Measure twice, cut once." Mergers will cost management time, board time, and considerable amounts of the organization's money. Depending on the size and complexity of the organization, six-figure costs are certain and seven figures a real possibility. (For instance, in February 2010, Care New England and Lifespan called off a proposed merger after spending $8 million and nearly three years going through the regulatory process.)[18] Even health systems that have considerable experience with mergers and acquisitions will at times need outside help from lawyers and consultants. The range of talent a merger may need also depends on the organization's size, the merger's complexity, and the experience of the parties in such transactions. The less experienced an organization, the more outside help it needs.

A danger to be avoided is to be tempted to cut corners—thereby saving money—because the merger appears to be straightforward and the leadership believes it has a handle on the proceedings (for example, believing no antitrust issues exist in a proposed merger). As one attorney reported, her colleague often responds to the price question of their services by saying, "You can pay me now, or pay me later,"[19] meaning it is wiser to invest up front in a properly conducted transaction than to ignore advice and face a more uncertain and higher cost when, down the road, the process does not result in the outcome planned.

With that caution in mind, it is important to distinguish between the value of preventive advisory services and repair services. *Price* for services is something you pay for once; *cost* is the money and time spent recovering from your mistakes. As one former large-system executive commented, mergers, acquisitions, and divestures are not part of the normal job for most executives, so hire professional help.[20]

Mergers are critical strategic options—options that will dictate your organization's future—so, once again, be sure to get the right talent in place early on. To paraphrase the carpenter, "measure twice, *pay* once."

Legal Considerations

Key legal issues frame any preparation for a merger. Areas that warrant special attention include confidentiality agreements, antitrust considerations, appropriate documentation, and the use of transaction and bond counsel.

Confidentiality Agreements

In short, bring in local counsel early. It is important that key leaders within the organization understand the importance and sensitivity of the matters under discussion. It is equally, if not more, important to be sure confidentiality agreements are executed upon entering discussion with another organization. This is a necessary first step once the parties decide discussions have merit in the context of the merger exploration. The hospital's or health system's internal or external legal counsel will be familiar with the steps required to protect the integrity of the respective parties and the process. It bears repetition: Counsel should be brought in early when a transaction is being contemplated.

Antitrust Considerations

Antitrust issues should be addressed at the outset when considering a merger or merger-like transaction. Transactions are treated like mergers for antitrust purposes if they involve a complete combination of the operations of the entities. This circumstance could occur through several legal forms, such as a change in corporate membership, formation of a partnership or contractual joint operating agreement, or acquisition of stock or assets.[21]

In this arena, it is critically important that health system or hospital executives and trustees understand certain precautions are in order. Until a transaction actually closes, the parties are considered competitors. The most important precaution for the negotiating parties is to *refrain from discussions* of the following:

- *Market share or service allocation.* Market share and market power are fundamental cornerstones of a position of power to influence pricing to the buyer of health care services, an antitrust red flag of glaring proportions.
- *Prices.* No discussion or exchange of information about pricing, or strategies around pricing (for instance, the ability to influence or benefit from managed care rates) should take place. Such discussion would be akin to two Realtors® getting together to discuss what commission they will charge their respective customers that come together over a real estate deal. This is collusion, and it is illegal.
- *Strategic plans.* No discussion or exchange of any non-public information should take place regarding an organization's strategic plan and the tactics supporting these plans.

Senior executives and trustees should note that several governmental authorities play important roles in a merger transaction, as their approval is often required. The Federal Trade Commission (FTC) is the most important federal authority in this discussion. The FTC's organization includes five commissioners, of whom no more than three can belong to the same political party.

Various departments within the FTC carry out the government's policies on trade and competition. The Bureau of Competition within the FTC reviews proposed hospital mergers for the potential impact on competition. (The U.S. Department of Justice, which in the past was also involved in rendering decisions on hospital mergers, tends now to review mergers relative to health insurance plans.)[22]

On the state level, executives should be aware of the views and past actions of the state's attorney general. Some have been very active in the matter of mergers, and you may be tempted to rely on your interpretation of their leanings, but no health care leader should ever take for granted the attorney general's likely view of your proposed merger.

The FTC does not distinguish between for-profit and not-for-profit entities. For-profit hospital companies, which frequently acquire, sell, or swap hospitals, usually are well versed in antitrust implications. Not-for-profit organizations, which tend to believe their transactions "benefit the community," often do not place antitrust issues near the top of their list of merger concerns and, as a result, are vulnerable to underestimating the need to engage antitrust counsel early in the process. This tendency is somewhat understandable, given the track record of unsuccessful government antitrust challenges against hospitals over the last ten to fifteen years. *However, it should be noted that this record of success is shifting toward the FTC's favor.*

In August 2007, some seven years *after* the transaction was consummated, the FTC ruled that Evanston Northwestern Healthcare's acquisition of Highland Park Hospital in the northern Chicago suburbs violated Section 7 of the Clayton Act. Having the benefit of seven years' worth of documentation post-merger, the FTC had at its disposal a record of activity on which to base its case. There was no question that prices were raised significantly following the merger; the dispute in this case related to the cause of the increase. The FTC prevailed, finding the price increases were the product of market power. The remedy was a change of conduct type rather than a divestiture, requiring Highland Park Hospital to negotiate managed care contracts separately from the other hospitals in the system.[23]

More recently, the FTC prevailed in 2008 in a challenge against Inova Health System, the large Fairfax, Virginia, health system, in its effort to merge Prince William Hospital of Manassas, Virginia, into its system. The FTC's concern was that a merger of Prince William into Inova Health System would have the effect of raising prices, as the FTC is watchful of smaller or unaffiliated entities joining larger systems to enjoy rate increases. Given Inova was a "must have" organization for health insurance plans, the FTC viewed the proposed merger as anti-competitive rather than pro-competitive.[24] (The government's guideline for analyzing market concentration is the Herfindahl-Hirschman Index [HHI], with high concentration considered a post-acquisition HHI exceeding a score of 1,800 and a change in the HHI as a result of the merger or acquisition greater than 50.)[25] The FTC prevailed when Inova dropped its pursuit of the merger, and ironically, as if to prove the FTC's concern, Prince William joined a health system located in another state.

Health care leaders should also note that the battle to capture outpatient revenues is on the radar screen of the FTC. In July 2009, the FTC challenged the 2008 acquisition of two outpatient centers by Carilion Clinic, contending that the acquisition left only two other freestanding outpatient centers in Roanoke, Virginia, a move the FTC contended eliminated necessary competition for the benefit of the consumer.[26] Carilion entered into a consent order with the FTC calling for the sale of the two centers to parties approved by the commission. Early in 2010, Carilion announced a buyer for one of the outpatient centers.[27]

The takeaway for health care executives is to understand that these cases, along with other non–health care cases, have bolstered the FTC's confidence and commitment to enforce federal laws and regulations regarding competition. The agency will look to foster the competitive tensions among hospitals, health insurance plans, and physicians that lend themselves to consumer choice and protection from predatory capability to raise prices.

In addition, executives should continue to follow the recent announcements by the Federal Trade Commission and the Department of Justice that they are contemplating a substantial rewrite of merger guidelines that date back to 1992. With the Obama administration's active enforcement philosophy, these developments will bear watching by health care leaders.[28]

Management is prudent when contemplating a transaction to require a preliminary antitrust analysis to assess the risk a transaction may present. Furthermore, placing the discussions and deliberations of an organization's proposed transaction under the protection of antitrust counsel is a wise consideration.

Documentation

Because market share and market power are chief determinants of market concentration in a proposed transaction, an organization's own documents tend to support its position. Go back through several years of strategic plans and slide shows in any hospital, and you will find sufficient information to define your organization's market share. It is hard to make a different case for market share when your own documents already tell the story.

What you write or say matters more than you think. What is written on note pads, sent in e-mails, or stated verbally is subject to scrutiny by outside organizations reviewing and approving or disapproving a merger transaction. Even transactions under legal protection of attorney-client privilege cannot undergo changes to documents, correspondence, and notes related to conversations made before the date of legal engagement. The lesson here, again, is to engage counsel early. If a merger does come under scrutiny, notes, files, dates, places, and names of people at meetings will all be part of such a review. Certain words, for example, raise red flags, such as *price, markets, eliminates,* and *allocations.* This scrutiny includes the work of consultants, which may either help or hurt your position. In the Evanston Northwestern case, the FTC found, based on the parties and their consultants' pre-merger documents, that they had three reasons for the merger: raising prices (bad), achieving economies of scale (good), and developing new programs (good). As one antitrust lawyer summarized the situation, "The moral of the story is clear: 'Bad' documents kill," and "good reasons for the merger and 'good' documents will not trump 'bad' reasons for the merger and 'bad' documents."[29]

Transaction Counsel

In addition to an organization's own legal counsel, another legal expert or team of experts that may be engaged is transaction counsel, who will help advise parties as to the risk, structure, and closing of the legal form of merger or affiliation. Transaction counsel is usually brought in by hospital counsel and can be jointly hired by multiple parties, in which case they work closely with the respective organizations' counsel. Sometimes they may be brought in late into the process, told by the CEOs of the organizations, for example, that "the deal is done, now make it happen."[30] Ideally, however, transaction counsel is brought in early in a pre-planning transaction.

Bond Counsel

Specialized counsel may be brought in pursuant to financing the transaction. For instance, bond counsel will represent the issuers of the bonds. They will render an opinion on the validity and tax exemption of the bonds being issued and review the transaction for compliance with Internal Revenue Service regulations.

Obtaining Government Approval for a Merger

Organizations that exceed thresholds of revenue or asset size in a proposed transaction are required by federal law to file a Hart-Scott-Rodino pre-merger notification. An organization's antitrust or transaction counsel will be familiar with these requirements. In addition, the requirements (dollar amount thresholds are adjusted annually for inflation) are spelled out on the FTC Web site (www.ftc.gov), readily available to the public. The FTC has thirty days to respond to a filing for merger approval. If it decides within that time to seek more information about the proposed merger, it will issue a "second request" for information. The second request is official notice that the government is requesting significantly more information and data with which it will deliberate in detail the competitive merits of the proposed transaction. This action is a red flag that the contemplated merger is falling under government scrutiny. Executives who have experienced a second request for additional information will confirm that the time and cost spent to comply takes on exponential proportions. For example, MaineHealth, in Portland, decided in late 2009 to cancel its deal with fifty-three-bed Goodall Hospital in Sanford, Maine, after the FTC made a second request for information, cost and time being factors in the decision.[31]

A merger not requiring a pre-merger notification can still come to the attention of the FTC from parties believed to be compromised competitively from a proposed transaction. For instance, an organization that is contemplating a merger by way of a joint operating agreement may fall outside the asset test thresholds requiring a notification filing, as assets are not merged in this legal model. However, complaints from managed care plans, physicians, unions, or employers can alert the FTC, commencing its involvement in a case, regardless of whether a Hart-Scott-Rodino notice is filed. The government particularly views managed care plans as a proxy for consumers.[32]

In addition to federal approvals, organizations need to comply with their state merger laws. For health system mergers covering multiple states, additional time and cost will be incurred to comply with the various laws. Again, an organization would be prudent to invest its time and money in doing its homework up front. Sound preparation and planning are key fundamentals to assess potential enterprise risk, time, and cost going forward.

Consultants

Larger health care systems often have substantial internal resources and thus limit the involvement of outside consultants. However, given that the organizations contemplating a merger are prohibited from exchanging certain strategic information until a transaction actually closes, third-party consultants are, at times, contracted to work with the parties as they move toward closing a transaction. As noted earlier in the antitrust discussion, it is important to choose consultants who are experienced and can work with multiple parties and their respective legal teams.

The following are various types of consultants and services that might be hired or used in a transaction, depending on size, complexity, and competitive market issues.

Financial adviser. Advises the client on financial merits of a transaction and/or advises as to other resources that might be needed to move the transaction toward close.

Business case consultant. Assists the organization(s) in making the business case for the transaction, often hired by both parties because they can review material the individual parties are not allowed to review. The product of their work tends to be a high-level analysis of the financial merits and risks of the proposed transaction.

Efficiency study. An analysis of the efficiencies and benefits that can only be derived from the merger, which can be developed by the same group of business case consultants. They work closely with, or are hired by, antitrust counsel when deemed necessary to conduct an efficiency study. These become important documents in seeking FTC and/or state government approval of a merger, as governmental authorities usually require projected efficiencies for the first five years of the merger.

Economist. Usually hired in conjunction with or by antitrust counsel, where the market dynamics of a proposed transaction and the risk of a challenge call for another set of experts to deal with the impact a merger may have on patient flow, market concentration, and pricing of services.

Valuation consultants. Hired when a determination needs to be made as to the amount or percentage of financial interest of the parties or the worth of assets needs to be valued.

Communication specialist. Some organizations, in contemplating the many internal and external stakeholders who need to be informed and brought along in a proposed transaction, will hire outside communication/crisis experts to help craft and guide the message, prepare responses to anticipated frequently asked questions, prepare for press announcements, and so on. Communication during the merger process is critical. Addressing why the organization is contemplating a merger, when it might happen, what the impact will be, and other questions requires agreement on who will speak for the organization and how often. Organizations must decide whether they have the talent internally or must hire expert help.

One executive with experience from several mergers noted that communication was the differentiator in well-managed merger processes. In citing her merger experiences between Hampton General and Sentara in Virginia, and another separate experience with Mary Immaculate in Virginia and Bon Secours Health System in Baltimore, both were characterized as organizations that communicated up front with employees and physicians on why a merger needed to be explored and the competitive environmental context that led to this decision. Though people naturally were concerned for their own future, upon consummation of these mergers, the communication process that was in place and the understanding of this information facilitated a smooth transition into the combined entities.[33]

Regardless of the decision to use internal or external resources (or a combination of the two), a communication plan is a must for all contemplated merger transactions.

Culture consultants. Given the critical issue of reconciling or creating a new culture in mergers, some organizations hire culture consultants to assist them in a pre-merger assessment of culture similarities and differences, or hire them post-merger to help bridge the many challenges that come into play in bringing two or more parties together. Culture is discussed in detail in chapter 4.

Other experts. Yes, even a few more outsiders may be brought to the transaction during the due diligence phase, mentioned later in this chapter.

Memorandum of Understanding/Letter of Intent

Once the health care entities agree on basic terms of the transaction, a memorandum of understanding (MOU) is drafted and signed by the parties. Sometimes this term is used interchangeably with the term *letter of intent.* This document sets forth the *preliminary* negotiated terms of the transaction, subject to further business and legal analysis.[34] The parties are still considered to be competitors at this point and as such still must ensure no anti-competitive actions take place. As a precursor to the definitive (final) agreement, the MOU is akin to getting engaged.

Business Plan: How Will We Run the Merged Organization?

Merger discussions lead to many questions, a few of which are cited in figure 3-6. Perhaps one of the more controversial debates about hospital mergers is when to prepare a business plan—before a transaction closes or after the deal is closed.

As one CEO relayed the story of his organization's mid-1990s merger, he stated there was no way the merger would have happened if the entities had had to develop a business plan before closing the transaction; however, looking back on a merger that failed within four years, he realized that the fact they could not work on a long-term vision and develop a business plan before close should have been a red flag. He further

Figure 3-6.   Questions That Typically Arise from Merger Discussions

- Will there be layoffs?
- What is the structure and hierarchy of the new organization?
- Do any services get consolidated, and if so, where? When?
- How and when do we implement identified merger efficiencies?
- What happens to employee benefits; how do we reconcile differences, and when?
- Do we keep ancillary departments at the same locations, or consolidate locations?
- Are there new services to invest in, especially where the community might be underserved?
- Do we form an obligated group for financing purposes?
- How do capital priorities and allocation get established?
- How do we pay for corporate overhead, and what is the allocation formula?
- Do we consolidate to one medical staff?
- Do we consolidate fund-raising organizations?
- What about information systems? When do we integrate? How do we reconcile cost versus benefits?
- What is our plan over the next three to five years?

commented that a business plan developed before close would have identified the issues that clearly doomed the merger a few years later, and perhaps the merger would not have been consummated in the first place.

This is precisely the point—a business plan developed *before* close will likely bring to the surface the difficult issues, and even hidden agendas. The organizations that can work through the difficult issues prior to closing and come up with a well-debated and -considered strategy are clearly on their way to a successful merger.

Returning to our case study of Progressive Health System, its preparation in determining why it wanted to merge and having clear merger objectives and screening criteria in place allowed it to quickly narrow eight interested parties down to two. One finalist was Progressive's longtime local competitor, the other a national "name" organization headquartered some 500 miles away. A business plan prepared with the help of outside consultants demonstrated that a transaction with the local competitor presented the greatest case for the benefit of the community in terms of operational cost savings, capital avoidance, improved access, and facilities coordination.

A few other examples of organizations that placed a premium on thoroughly understanding the business aspects of a merger before closing include those highlighted in the following paragraphs.

Catholic Healthcare West (CHW) Chief Financial Officer Mike Blaszyk chairs that organization's Transition Committee, which oversees merger and acquisition opportunities, and insists on a business plan up front in a transaction. He admits this requirement sometimes resulted in lost deals, but as part of the value and criteria of CHW's mergers and acquisitions, it gives the organization the ability to walk away from deals itself.[35]

The formation in 1996 of BayCare Health System pursuant to a business plan developed before the close of the transaction served to focus nine hospitals on a common vision with a business plan and metrics to measure performance for the initial five years of the joint operating agreement.

Recently, Upper Chesapeake Health, a two-hospital system in Harford County, Maryland, sent out a request for proposals for merger partners, insisting on, as part of its objectives and criteria, a multiple-staged transaction prior to close. The key pre-closing phases center on a business plan with agreement on financial resources for clinical services development along with a plan related to facility development and/or replacement. The University of Maryland Health System agreed to enter into this planned merger partnership with Upper Chesapeake Health, in which both parties will need to agree on the business plan before the merger is consummated, scheduled for 2013.[36]

Avoiding difficult issues prior to close will not make them any easier to deal with after closing a merger. Organizations that cannot reach agreement on difficult issues during the negotiating phase should see this obstacle as a warning as to the merits of the proposed transaction. Thus, the process of how to get the merger done and linking it back to merger objectives calls for development of a business plan before closing. It either aligns most critical issues or exposes differences that must be reconciled if the merger indeed has merit to the parties and to the communities they serve. Developing a business plan is just one of the steps, summarized in figure 3-7, to guide organizations through a merger.

Definitive Agreement: The Deal Is Finalized

Once agreement is reached on the business merits of the proposed deal, a definitive agreement (sometimes called *master*

Figure 3-7. How to Get through the Merger Process

- Inform/engage your own counsel.
- Obtain signed confidentiality agreements from negotiating entities.
- Assess antitrust considerations and engage transaction counsel.
- Develop a communication plan and identify spokespersons.
- Prepare a preliminary business case and engage outside consultants as necessary.
- Sign a letter of intent upon agreement on the merits of the business case.
- Commence preliminary due diligence.
- Prepare a detailed business plan (which could serve as an efficiency study if required for antitrust purposes).
- Sign the definitive agreement upon final approval of the transaction.
- Complete due diligence and final legal/regulatory filings.

agreement) is signed, setting forth the rights and obligations of the parties in the transaction.[37] This document is, in essence, the marriage contract, a binding agreement.

Progressive Health System encountered delays in reaching a definitive agreement due to antitrust challenges that it, and particularly its larger partner, had underestimated. The government filed a second request for information that delayed the closing by months and added considerable cost. However, the board and management of both parties felt strongly that the merger objectives presented high value to the communities they served and as such were critical to getting the deal done. From the time Progressive first contemplated the "why merge?" question to working through the process of understanding what it brought to the table in terms of strengths and weaknesses, finalizing its objectives, defining its criteria, and negotiating its preferred deal, a period of eighteen months had passed, with the final six months spent dealing with the antitrust investigation. Its perseverance paid off, and an excellent management team along with a dedicated board made this mid-1990s merger a success, ongoing now for sixteen years, with Progressive's original merger objectives having been more than sufficiently met.

Due Diligence

The due diligence process involves disclosure of pertinent information by each party before a transaction can be closed formally and legally. Preliminary due diligence starts early in the process and is completed upon or shortly after the signing of the definitive agreement.

Though many tend to think of due diligence as a legal process, the business component of this step is probably more important than the legal component,[38] given the need to review financials, the physical plant, the clinical services, medical staff credentialing, union contracts, and so on. Due diligence is an investigative process performed by attorneys, accountants, and consultants. Based on the findings of this process, human resources consultants (reviewing and reconciling compensation and benefit policies); environmental, or "green," experts (assessing environmental hazards and risk); real estate appraisers (assessing land and real estate holdings); and others could become part of the due diligence team depending on the substance and complexity of issues that surfaced at the outset of the due diligence process.

In addition, sometimes a *fairness opinion* may be required. A fairness opinion is an analysis of the financial aspects of the deal from the point of view of one or more parties to the transaction. It is usually requested by a board or governmental entity. Such an opinion may provide an extra layer of fiduciary responsibility, but it is not a substitute for sound business judgment. Fairness opinions have become controversial because of perceived conflicts of interest with the financial adviser or accountant executing them.

Finally, transaction counsel and the organizations' respective counsel will assist management in making required final regulatory and governmental filings.

Conclusion: The End Is the Beginning

One executive spoke on behalf of the many who have been through a merger process when she stated that, by this time, exhaustion has long set in.[39] A process that commenced with "why merge?" and evolved into "what do we want out of a merger?" (objectives and criteria), requiring an inordinate amount of management and board time along with that of an array of attorneys and consultants, brings us not to the end, but merely to the beginning. The goal moving forward is to make good on the objectives, merits, and efficiencies of the transaction, which must translate into better access to care, improved competitive cost of care, and renewed focus on the quality of care rendered in our hospitals.

References

1. Bruce Japsen, "Another Record Year for Dealmaking," *Modern Healthcare* (December 23, 1996): 40.
2. Deanna Bellandi, "Spinoffs, Big Deals Dominate in '99," *Modern Healthcare* (January 10, 2000): 38.
3. Sandy Lutz, "1995: A Record Year for Hospital Deals," *Modern Healthcare* (December 18, 1995): 46.
4. Japsen, "Another Record Year," 40.
5. Patrick Reilly, "Mergers Minus the Mania," *Modern Healthcare* (January 20, 2003): 38.
6. Melanie Evans and Vince Galloro, "M&A Trend: No Big Deal," *Modern Healthcare* (January 21, 2008): 24.
7. Lutz, "1995," 50.
8. Bellandi, "Spinoffs," 42.
9. Sandy Lutz, "Let's Make a Deal," *Modern Healthcare* (December 19, 1994): 49.
10. Lutz, "1995," 46.
11. Bruce Japsen, "An Off Year for Consolidation," *Modern Healthcare* (January 12, 1998): 48.
12. Vince Galloro and Jeff Tieman, "Hitting the Brakes," *Modern Healthcare* (January 14, 2002): 31.
13. Deanna Bellandi, "The Deals Are Off," *Modern Healthcare* (January 8, 2001): 44.
14. Galloro and Tieman, "The Deals Are Off," 24.
15. Lutz, "Let's Make a Deal," 52.
16. James Thornton, former CEO, Brandywine Hospital, telephone interview with author, July 21, 2009.
17. Patricia A. Cahill and Maryanna Coyle, *Catholic Health Initiatives, a Spirit of Innovation, a Legacy of Care, the Early Years* (Denver: Catholic Health Initiatives, 2006), 39.
18. Felice J. Freyer, "Issues That Prompted Failed Hospital Merger Remain," *Providence Journal* (March 1, 2010).
19. Toby Singer, attorney, Jones Day, interview with author, Washington, D.C., July 6, 2009.
20. Jerry P. Widman, former CEO, Ascension Health, interview with author, Dawsonville, Georgia, October 8, 2009.
21. David A. Ettinger and Stanford P. Berenbaum, *Health Care Mergers and Acquisitions: The Antitrust Perspective.* BNA's Health Law

& Business Series. (Washington, D.C.: Bureau of National Affairs, 1996), 1400.01.C.

22. Singer interview.

23. Jeff Miles, "Observations and Lessons from the FTC's Evanston Northwestern Healthcare Hospital-Merger Decision," *The Health Lawyer*, 20, no. 1 (October 2007), 24.

24. Toby Singer, attorney, Jones Day, and Matt Reilly, assistant director, Bureau of Competition, Federal Trade Commission, separate interviews with author, Washington, D.C., July 6, 2009, and August 26, 2009, respectively.

25. Ettinger and Berenbaum, *Health Care Mergers*, 1400.05.B.2.

26. Federal Trade Commission, *FTC Challenges Carilion's Acquisition of Outpatient Medical Clinics* (Washington D.C.: Federal Trade Commission), 1 [http://www.ftc.gov/opa/2009/07/carilion.shtm]. Accessed August 31, 2009.

27. Gregg Blesch, "Carilion Finds a Taker," *Modern Healthcare* (February 1, 2010): 12.

28. Gregg Blesch, "Rethinking the Rules," *Modern Healthcare* (September 28, 2009): 10.

29. Miles, "Observations and Lessons," 26.

30. Stuart Lockman, attorney, Honigman & Miller, telephone interview with author, August 6, 2009.

31. Vince Galloro and Joe Carlson, "Ready for a Resurgence," *Modern Healthcare* (January 18, 2010): 28.

32. Singer interview.

33. Phyllis Stoneburner, RN, chief nursing officer, Obici Hospital, Sentara Health, interview with author, Suffolk, Virginia, December 4, 2009.

34. American Hospital Association, "Glossary of Hospital and Health Care System Merger, Acquisition and Consolidation Terms" (Chicago: American Hospital Association, 1989, 3).

35. Michael D. Blaszyk, chief financial officer, Catholic Healthcare West, telephone interview with author, July 15, 2009.

36. Rachel Konopacki, "Hospitals Join University," *The Aegis*, no. 53 (July 3, 2009): 1–2.

37. American Hospital Association, "Glossary," 3.

38. John Swartz, attorney, Sisters of St. Francis Health System, telephone interview with author, August 17, 2009.

39. Ruth W. Brinkley, RN, FACHE, president and CEO, Carondelet Health Network, Ascension Health, interview with author, Washington, D.C., November 13, 2009.

4

What about Those Culture Issues?

Culture will eat strategy. A cliché, perhaps, but the reality is that executives in any industry know that poor culture fit will compromise strategy in whole or in part. Every business, hospital, and health system has a culture. In a merger, unresolved culture conflicts can cripple or terminate a merger. One former chief medical officer observed that his newly merged organization was characterized by culture conflicts that reminded him of "a steel cage match," bringing to mind the antics of televised professional wrestling.

In their book *Corporate Culture*, Deal and Kennedy quote a definition of culture as the "integrated pattern of human behavior that includes thought, speech, action and artifacts and depends on man's capacity for learning and transmitting knowledge to succeeding generations."[1] Perhaps a shorter, more common, version will do: "the way we do things around here."

PROMINA Health System of Atlanta was named the number one integrated health system by *Hospitals & Health Networks* in 1998.[2] The system's chief executive officer (CEO), Bernie Brown, gained national recognition, as did the organization's model of integration. A few years later, this system folded and no longer exists. How does a health system go from being number one nationally to being defunct in a few short years?

Formed in 1994, this not-for-profit system had five subsystems and at its peak consisted of thirteen hospitals and more than 2,000 physicians. Its compelling reason for formation was to improve the founding organization's competitive position for managed care contracting, particularly following the joint venture of Emory University Hospital with the for-profit Columbia Healthcare System. It is Brown's view that mergers happen because people either like each other or have a common enemy[3]—PROMINA had both. The CEOs of the founding subsystems knew each other; it was an affiliation built on relationships.[4] All but one of PROMINA's hospitals were part of a hospital authority, so the idea of a merger of assets was not part of its thinking. PROMINA's leadership thought the affiliation gave the system the best of both worlds: a virtual merger (with its potential benefits of economies of scale) and autonomy.

Culture differences were not viewed as significant. In fact, one exercise conducted by Brown involved laying out the mission, vision, and value statements from all the system's organizations, and they proved to be amazingly similar. This test provided additional comfort to a number of board members.[5]

In his book, *Lessons Learned on the Way Down* (United Writers Press, 2007), Brown details what he saw as the reasons for the demise of PROMINA. Clearly, a few of the compelling reasons that drove the group to come together were no longer relevant, as the Emory-HCA joint venture did not last. In addition, a number of the PROMINA hospitals that were strong financially felt they were contributing more to the system than they were receiving. Thus, shared power became an issue, and the lack of full integration made it relatively easy to consider exiting the merger. Personalities and individual values clashed and eroded commitment among institutional leaders. An additional layer of management for the organization's system was seen as a bureaucracy, which some leaders considered burdensome.

Finally, culture differences, which did not seem so important at first, became more significant as PROMINA evolved. In Brown's view, the foregoing reasons were but components of one overarching cause, which centered on the concept of system "value." According to Brown, "the hard lesson that I gained from this is that no enterprise will survive and flourish in the long run unless it brings real as well as perceived value to those it serves." Several years after Brown's retirement, "This organization, which we once viewed as our salvation, was laid to rest without fanfare or ceremony."[6]

If PROMINA ended in fractional relationships, perhaps a contrasting situation can be found in Catholic Health East (CHE), based in Newtown Square, Pennsylvania, a suburb of Philadelphia. Retired CEO Robert Stanek cites culture as the key to CHE's success in carrying out its mission. This system was formed in 1997 from a merger of three systems involving eleven congregations and twenty-five hospitals along the East Coast. He described the merger formation as "made in heaven." The sponsors' singular focus of forming a competitive Catholic system to carry out its mission was foremost on their minds. Stanek states that the easiest part of his job is working with the sponsors because of their total commitment to making CHE work.

According to Stanek, CHE's culture is "relational" and "participative." As the system CEO, he judges his own success by the number of unilateral decisions he does *not* have to make. In maintaining the CHE culture, the role of the local boards is deemed very important, given the system's local orientation toward health care. The local board's role is part of the "relational culture" of CHE. Stanek describes the reserve powers of the system as being similar to those of other systems, but where they differ is how words and actions become important components of building a relational and participative culture. For instance, local boards have "preliminary approval" responsibility rather than being charged with merely "making recommendations," while the system maintains final approval for its areas of designated authority. To further assist in building a relational and participative culture of understanding between local and system responsibilities, about 65 percent of all CHE system committees are staffed by local board members, with the understanding that in their capacity of participating on these committees they represent the system, rather than their local hospital. Stanek sees this cross-fertilization as an important contributing factor in the ability to build comprehensive understanding across the system, thus providing dividends to the working relationship and appreciation of roles between local and system initiatives.

Understanding one's own organizational culture helped CHE to successfully integrate five hospitals it acquired in 2001 from another Catholic system with a different culture. Furthermore, understanding one's own culture allows leadership to know when to walk away from merger or acquisition opportunities with organizations whose culture differences do not merit the risk of going forward with such a transaction.[7]

Defining Corporate Culture

What factors determine the type of culture a hospital or health system has? Deal and Kennedy describe five key elements in their research on corporate cultures:

- Business environment
- Values
- Heroes
- Rites and rituals
- Culture network/communication

Business environment. Each organization faces a different reality in the market depending on the depth and breadth of its services, competitors, customers, technology, regulatory influence, and so forth. The environment in which a health system or hospital operates determines what it must do to succeed. For instance, the threat of for-profit hospital encroachment and having to deal with big insurance companies in a competitive managed care environment fostered not-for-profit hospitals to come together and protect not-for-profit health care. The business environment is the single greatest influence in shaping corporate culture.

Values. These include basic concepts and beliefs of an organization that form the heart of the corporate culture. Perhaps our faith-based hospitals and health systems embody their values most openly. Yet not all faith-based mergers are successful, even when they are of organizations affiliated with the same faith, so it takes more than values to achieve a common culture. Nevertheless, values are a critical component of culture and help define success for employees and business associates. Organizations with strong common values have established a standard of achievement by which their leaders talk openly and without embarrassment about the beliefs.

Heroes. Heroes in this context personify the culture values and provide tangible role models for others to follow. These achievers are known to virtually every employee and show "what you have to do to succeed around here." One thinks of Robert Cathcart, the retired CEO of Pennsylvania Hospital, who upon his retirement in the early 1990s was only the third CEO *of the century* at his organization. This fact, among other reasons, is why he is known as "Mr. Hospital."

Rites and rituals. The systematic, planned routines and rituals of day-to-day life in our hospitals and health systems demonstrate to stakeholders the kind of behavior expected within the organization. Various ceremonies (employee service recognition, doctors' day, nurses' week, annual celebrations, religious ceremonies, and so on) provide visible and potent examples of what the organization stands for.

Culture network/communication. The informal but primary "carriers" of communication within an organization disseminate the corporate values and heroic mythology. These are the storytellers, priests, and whisperers who form a hidden hierarchy of power; learning to tap this network effectively is an ideal way to achieve culture-related goals and understand what is going on throughout the organization.[8] Even in organizations with dysfunctional leadership, the informal leaders know what work-arounds are required to get things done.

In the period of hospital merger mania in the 1990s, the late, great business author Peter Drucker wrote that changing corporate culture had become the latest management fad.[9] One health care executive described an experience he had had just a few years ago while interviewing for the CEO position at the flagship hospital of a newly merged organization composed of two faith-based entities of different religious affiliations. While spending the day on-site interviewing with various people and making rounds throughout the campus, the candidate asked everyone he met what barriers impeded the organization's progress; the consistent answer given was, "We can't figure out what our culture is." At the summation conference at the end of a long day of interviews, the candidate was asked for his overall thoughts. He responded that he was no longer a candidate for the job. When someone from the stunned group asked why, the candidate responded, "The leadership of the organization does not make decisions—that *is* your culture!" He succinctly identified the organization's formal definition of culture as being camouflage for the actual culture, which was defined by a lack of decision making, action, and accountability.

Board/Sponsors' Impact on Merged Cultures

The board of the newly formed organization and any sponsors involved play a significant role in the development of a cohesive culture throughout the entity. The scenarios that follow illustrate the board's and sponsor's impact on culture.

When the Deal Lacks Clarity or Commitment

In 1998, St. Mary's Hospital of the Palatine Health System and Cabell Hospital, both of Huntington, West Virginia, decided to merge after decades of fierce competition. The physical distance between these two hospitals is three miles, approximately a seven-minute drive.

The compelling forces of this merger were the presence of managed care, for-profit encroachment, and competition from larger regional competitors, both in and out of state. The two hospitals also asked a smaller hospital, Pleasant Valley, in Point Pleasant, West Virginia, to join. Being smaller, Pleasant Valley did not want to appear to have been taken over, and the three parties agreed to a merger of equal representation. The two Huntington hospitals, the key players in the merger, were viewed as having complementary strengths, with St. Mary's enjoying a good reputation in heart and cancer care and Cabell being recognized for its high-quality pediatric and obstetric care. The challenge for the merger was the culture differences. How would they overcome the many years of intense competition between them? No CEO was selected at the inception of the merger; instead, the three hospital CEOs ran their respective operations, and any system decision required the unanimous vote of all three. The board was composed of an equal number of representatives from all three organizations, and the parent board had reserve powers over budget and financial matters.

Though the board was not empowered to obligate the hospitals, it could move money around within the system; this power would later prove to be a litmus test for the system. The cultures were very different, with St. Mary's being Catholic and having a long tenure in the community and Cabell being seen as a semi-public type of hospital. At one time, its board was appointed by commissioners and was unionized.

Mike Sellards, CEO of the smaller Pleasant Valley Hospital, observed the two Huntington hospitals attempting to merge. He noticed how difficult it was for people who were fiercely competitive to suddenly work together. "Hi, I am your friend, I am here to help," did not sell well in the early stages of the merger.

After two years, the CEO of Cabell decided to retire, and the board named Tom Jones, then CEO of St. Mary's, as the CEO of the three-hospital system. Jones was sensitive to St. Mary's differences with Cabell and made numerous attempts to address them as they surfaced. One such situation revolved around Cabell Hospital's desire for a cardiac catheterization laboratory. Jones, with the agreement of the leadership team, hired an independent consultant to evaluate this need. Jones believed that St. Mary's (his legacy organization) would get the cath lab, but the consultant recommended that Cabell receive it. Jones reports that time eventually proved this assessment to be the correct business and patient care decision and believed Cabell felt good about the process used to reach this recommendation.

Similarly, when the decision was to be made about choosing a group purchasing organization (GPO), an independent consultant was hired to make a recommendation. Prior to the merger, each hospital had used a different GPO. The consultant recommended the GPO used by St. Mary's. Cabell joined this purchasing organization, and as Jones points out, after the merger later broke up, they continued operating under the same GPO, seemingly validating the soundness of this business decision.

In another ironic, if not humorous, culture difference, Jones noted early in his role as new system CEO that Cabell had a full-time chaplain on staff. At a meeting, he asked the chaplain if he would offer a prayer or reflection (common at Catholic hospitals), thinking this act would be a culture builder. He later received a letter from someone in attendance at the meeting advising him not to try to turn Cabell into a Catholic hospital, the letter stating, "We don't pray over here."

Furthermore, the culture building involved picking a new corporate name to brand the system, and the name "Genesis" came from a Cabell board member. The name later evolved to Genesis Hospital System.

Despite these attempts by management to build a culture from two different and previously competing organizations, the merger came apart four years after its inception. In considering a hospital acquisition opportunity that presented itself to Genesis Hospital System, the sisters representing St. Mary's apparently believed the ability of the system board to "move money around" to finance the proposed transaction was ceding more control than they desired. Jones, along with a key board member, Mike Perry, was called into a meeting one morning, at which the sisters informed them they wanted out of the merger. The exit clause that had been placed into the original agreement—one that no one thought would ever be used, given the seemingly prohibitive price to exit—was invoked.[10,11]

As Mike Perry, a former banker and well-respected hospital trustee, observed, "[Genesis] did not break up due to failure; maybe it broke up because it was going to be successful."[12] Another key executive summarized the entire situation: "We could not find a way to solve the culture issues."

The merger, formed in 1998, ended in 2002.

When the Board "Gets It" (and Is Ahead of Management)

In contrast to the board's role in the Huntington experience was that of the board in the Alta Bates (part of Sutter Health) merger with Summit Medical Center in 1999. The cultures were very different: Alta Bates saw its organization as slightly below academic medical center status, while Summit, located in downtown Oakland, California, was viewed by Sutter to have a "victim" mentality. The cultures of the medical staff were also very different—the fact that they are still separate ten years after the merger indicates the scale of the difference. However, the event that triggered the genesis of a new culture occurred when the new capital budget was presented to the board shortly after the merger was consummated. Alta Bates's former CEO, Warren Kirk, now chief operating officer (COO) of the merged entity, presented his legacy Alta Bates hospital budget to the board even though Summit's financial information was not yet available for review. When the board understood that only partial budget information was being presented, Kirk was told to bring back one systemwide budget. The message was unmistakably clear—the board was of one mind, and it expected to operate as one organization, albeit with multiple delivery sites. From this time on, all financials are presented as one, not even broken out by campus.

When Kirk later took over as system CEO of the merged Alta Bates Summit, the merger process presented a sudden, serious financial crisis. He candidly admitted he did not have much time to think about culture. However, the urgency of the financial challenge related to pulling the merger together forced people to collaborate, so through the crisis they were slowly building an Alta Bates Summit culture.[13] Having survived this crisis in 2002, the merged entity has gone on to enjoy sound operational performance throughout the remainder of the decade.

When the Board Takes the Long-Term View and Builds Trust

On Florida's eastern coast in the mid-1990s, Holmes Regional Medical Center, looking to merge in response to growing competition from medical groups, managed care plans, and for-profit entities, decided to partner with Cape Canaveral Hospital. With a threefold size disparity in favor of Holmes, the CEO of Holmes and its board offered Cape Canaveral 50 percent of the board seats. This gesture was not offered just to be nice; the board took a long-term view that as members of not-for-profit organizations they had a fiduciary responsibility to share the management of health care services and resources in Brevard County, and size and egos were not to get in the way. The hospitals' boards agreed that the first board chair would come from Holmes, the second from Cape Canaveral, and this agreement was not even put in writing. The board chairs continue to rotate to this day, as the seeds of trust demonstrated by the original CEOs and board leadership planted a culture that continues fifteen years into this successful merger.[14]

When the Board Structure or Sponsorship Involves Merging Multiple Cultures

In contemplating the formation of Catholic Health Initiatives (CHI) (formed in 1996), the founding sponsors were deeply committed to developing a national Catholic system in response to a changing health care environment. They were aware the three founding sponsors had three different cultures. The Franciscan Health System (Philadelphia) was viewed as centralized, the Catholic Healthcare Corporation (Omaha, Nebraska) was viewed as decentralized, and the Sisters of Charity (Cincinnati, Ohio) was thought to be somewhere in the middle. The sponsors' ideal was to take the best of each, but in terms of culture and operating model, they did not want either the centralized or decentralized model.[15] Instead, the sponsors established a new framework for the kind of organizational culture they desired.

Values and Their Impact on Mergers

In the urgency to respond to environmental and market challenges, organizations at times rush to get a merger transaction completed, sometimes skimming over the differences in corporate values between organizations. Perhaps the thinking is that these issues can be worked out later. Let us review a few cases that provide lessons on appreciating the importance of understanding corporate values.

Academics and Research versus Full-Time Employed Physicians

Conflict over the cultures consistent with academic/research physicians and hospital-employed physicians arose with the merger of Hershey Medical Center and Geisinger Health System in Pennsylvania in 1997. At the time, both organizations were viewed as financially healthy, but both endorsed the environmental prognostications that local hospitals and physician groups would consolidate into large health systems in response to perceived financial threats that would challenge access to capital and managed care competitive positions. Though news reports quoted a key executive as saying the cultures between the two organizations would be the merged entity's strength, the reality pointed to a different picture. It was reported that "Hershey Medical Center's style of collective governance by cooperating with independent and strong academic departments clashed with Geisinger's style of managing full-time, salaried physicians in a multispecialty group practice."[16]

In addition, independent physicians not associated with the Penn State Geisinger Health Plan did not support the merger, believing the real purpose was to secure profits and restrict choice. They resisted expectations to refer patients to the two organizations or to its health plan.

The dissolution of the merger was announced in November 1999, just two years after its consummation. The cultural differences were viewed as a significant factor, the differences between the two having been underestimated. "Any organization possesses unique and immeasurable history, informal yet important relational networks, management styles, local opinion leaders, and institutional pride that can be easily underestimated in business plans but may act as powerful determinants of the success or failure of any merger."[17]

Perhaps, as Jaan Sidorov, MD, writes, "a corollary lesson may be that senior leaders caught up in the heady enthusiasm of a potential merger may be less able to objectively assess the suitability of their respective organizations' cultures."[18] This lesson in objectivity is a critical point worth deliberating for management and boards seeking merger partners.

When Faith Cannot Transcend Inherent Value Differences

One executive, experienced in more than a half dozen mergers, summed up his entire tenure as trying to bring together two faith-based organizations of different religious orientation. Let us call the entity St. Hope, a merger of two large hospitals, one Catholic and one Protestant affiliated.

The merger, consummated almost ten years ago, has struggled since its inception to realize its potential. The compelling reason for the merger was to obtain a significant increase in market share. However, the culture clashes between the organizations were viewed by this executive as so severe that it caused tremendous internal tension, compromising strategic initiatives that competitors took advantage of, such as hiring away key physicians and groups and preventing the organization from building on its existing clinical strengths. This inability, of course, is a violation of one of the five deadly business sins expounded by Drucker: "slaughtering tomorrow's opportunity on the altar of yesterday."[19] When the former CEO was asked if, in hindsight, this merger really made sense, his immediate reaction was, "No." The one hospital that enjoyed a considerable strength in cardiology should have spent its time and money building this strength rather than compromising its competitive position over the years to make a merger work. Since this executive left four years ago, the organization has seen another turnover in the CEO position, further highlighting this merger's struggle.

As one writer described business deals, "there are clean deals and dirty deals. Clean deals have clear constituent pieces, are easy to bring together and line up, and carry few or surmountable obstacles. Dirty deals have deep complications, broad variables, proliferating unknowns. With a dirty deal there's potential profit but much mess—to much underbrush, no clear path."[20] This faith-based merger resulting in the organization we call St. Hope would seem to be a dirty deal.

The 1994 merger of New Orleans of Mercy and Baptist, discussed in chapter 3, provides another example in which faith orientation does not always translate to faith-aligned values. The merged organization, which one year later was acquired by Tenet Healthcare Corporation, saw culture differences that led Tenet to run the two hospitals as separate entities, each with its own management team.[21]

Faith-based merger partners need to pay attention to culture issues as much as any other organization. As a New Testament verse says, "Faith by itself, if it is not accompanied by action, is dead."[22]

When Leaders Take Time to Understand
Each Other's Values

P. Terrence O'Rourke, MD, was the first board chair of the merger formed between Catholic hospitals sponsored by the Sisters of Charity out of Cincinnati and Porter Care hospitals sponsored by Adventist Health System. Today these entities are known as Centura, a joint venture hospital company sponsored by Catholic Health Initiatives and Adventist. O'Rourke believes one aspect of the merger approached correctly early on was spending significant time attempting to understand each other's culture and values.

The Adventist culture emphasized prevention and healthy lifestyles, while the Catholic system focused on care of the underserved and poor. However, time spent at retreats and board meetings proved that both parties had values that were more similar than different.

The two organizations agreed that the hospitals forming this joint venture would continue their identity and culture with respect to their organizational legacies. With that, the culture ground rules had been established.[23]

Whether or not this approach is the best for other organizations, it is clear this organization deliberated the changes it could and could not endorse. Unless a compelling vision and reason exist for making a change, winning people over to a new way of operating will prove difficult. The change contemplated needs to be an improvement on the current state.

One basic principle of executive coaching is to understand what it takes to make significant change. This principle involves answering the following questions:

- What are the benefits of maintaining the status quo?
- What does the organization lose if the patterns are changed?
- What will be the specific benefits of making the change?

- Do the benefits of the change supersede the benefits of maintaining the status quo?

Joe Swedish, CEO of Trinity Health, in Novi, Michigan, having served in both for-profit and not-for-profit organizations, notes that, in his experience, bringing two mature organizations together is the toughest challenge, as there is no burning platform to advance change.[24]

Pat Shehorn, CEO of Resurrection Health Care's Westlake Hospital and West Suburban Medical Center, in suburban Chicago, stated the positive side of the motivation coin well when she said she learned from a former boss that "sufficient dissatisfaction plus clear vision equals a brighter future."[25]

The CEO as Cornerstone of Successfully Merged Cultures

When we talk about merging, changing, or forming a new culture pursuant to a merger, what we are really speaking to is changing behavior.

As Drucker viewed it, culture is singularly persistent, and changing behavior works only if the process can be based on the existing culture.[26] In his view, changes to habits are needed, not changes to the culture. The first step is to define what results are needed to make a merger a success. Second, consider where within your own systems these results have been achieved already.[27] The CEOs who understand this are in a position to have a powerful impact on their organization and market.

Merging Previously Fierce Competitors

The merger of Morton Plant Hospital, in Clearwater, Florida, with the two-hospital system Mease Health Care, in Dunedin, Florida, three miles north of Clearwater, in 1994 joined two previously fierce competitors. In fact, Mease was in existence because a former Morton Plant physician, Jack Mease, decided to start a hospital at the request of the citizens of Dunedin. The hospital opened in 1937, and after more than five decades of competition, the board decided the right thing for the community was to merge with the competing organization. The cultures, however, were very different; Morton Plant was viewed as the 800-pound arrogant guerrilla, while Mease was viewed as the smaller underdog. Former CEO Frank Murphy (now retired), in the spirit of building culture throughout Morton Plant Mease by changing behavior, focused the merger integration around four key areas: leadership, communication, recognition and reward, and patient outcomes education and training.

Leadership

Murphy first decided he would work as a partner with the CEO of Mease, Phil Beauchamp, who was named COO of the system. Clearly only one CEO was in place, but Murphy wanted to present a united front to stakeholders. So he created the "office of the president" and moved his office to the Mease Dunedin campus, where Beachamp was located. This move alone made a significant statement. Both Murphy and Beauchamp were named to the new system board. As they worked closely together, trust grew with each action step.

Second, a new management team, down to the department head level, was selected within sixty days. This task was important because the merger became subject to an antitrust consent decree blocking full merger for ten years. A leadership team was needed that was committed to making this deal work when a consent decree could have easily become an excuse to undo the transaction.

The core of the behavior change was Murphy's focus on continuous quality improvement (CQI), a concept he had studied and committed to as a process to improve patient care. Murphy and Beauchamp conducted more than a hundred town hall meetings with stakeholders to instill the CQI philosophy. The working mantra and culture focus for the new organization became "Service, Cost, Outcomes." Murphy taught the CQI principles to his managers, who then became disciples to teach others in the organization. In the mold of Drucker, Murphy defined the needed results of the merger and built it on the good qualities and processes that were already in place within the member entities.

Communication

The focus on communication led the leadership to examine all modes of communication at each organization—the words and methods used to reach the hospital staff and the community. The vice presidents led task forces of employees to help define the values of the newly joined organization. For instance, the term *team member* replaced the word *employee*, and a video was produced titled "I am Morton Plant Mease."

After about three years, team members began to feel and function as one organization.

Recognition and Reward

Everyone involved with the organization has a stake in improving the service, cost structure, and patient care outcomes. Team members are honored at annual award ceremonies for achievements based on their contributions to meeting or exceeding key performance indicators. Gift certificates are periodically awarded during the year to recognize actions supporting organizational values. And recognition in various in-house publications helps reinforce corporate goals and acknowledge team members' achievements.

Patient Outcomes Education and Training

With physicians and team members working together, the focus in this key area was to reduce variation of patient outcomes, starting with high-volume and high-cost areas. The CEO led and set the tone for the importance of the focus on patient outcomes, working closely with the chief medical officer and the medical staff leadership.

This behavior and metrics focus has resulted in two of the three Pinellas County–based Morton Plant Mease hospitals enjoying annual selection as top 100 hospitals in one or more areas of clinical service.[28]

Building a Culture Based on Partnership

An important postscript to building a culture by focusing behavior on the results that need to be achieved occurred two years later when Morton Plant Mease joined what became known as the BayCare Health System, which consists of nine hospitals in the Tampa Bay area functioning under a joint operating agreement.

BayCare was formed in large part as a response to the significant encroachment of for-profit health care taking place in Florida. The objective of the merger was to preserve community-owned (not-for-profit) health care. Frank Murphy became CEO of this system, with revenues of more than $1 billion when it formed in 1996. He used the same principles across the system to form a new management team within sixty days, reducing management from fifty-two vice presidents down to twenty-three. (At that time, Beauchamp became CEO of Morton Plant Mease). Rather than create a large central office for the system, Murphy broke the organization into three community health alliances serving the three major cities of Tampa, St. Petersburg, and Clearwater, a mechanism by which the organization could be responsive to local boards and communities. The CQI process was rolled out across the system, building on those areas that were already performing effectively. These initial actions formed a solid foundation for success that BayCare Health System continues to enjoy fifteen years later.[29]

Craig Brethauer, vice president (VP) of Human Resources at BayCare, had a unique view of these two mergers, having started at Mease heading up the human resources department then becoming VP of Human Resources of the combined

Morton Plant Mease and later for the BayCare system. He describes Murphy's accomplishment as having successfully built a culture based on partnership, where all involved felt they had a stake in the merged organization, while respecting the legacy organizations. Brethauer's view is that the Morton Plant Mease culture jelled fairly quickly, while the larger and more complex BayCare system (two Catholic hospitals, one Baptist hospital, and the others not-for-profit secular hospitals) probably took closer to ten years to become "BayCare."[30]

Merging Physician and Hospital Cultures: Building a Culture of Action and Trust

In the early 1990s, two San Francisco hospitals, Pacific Medical Center and Children's Medical Center, merged. They each brought a different culture to the new entity. Pacific Medical Center enjoyed a culture of teaching with an orientation to academic medicine, while Children's physicians considered themselves the "real doctors." The merged organization became known as California Pacific Medical Center (CPMC).

The leadership brought in a facilitator to help merge the medical staff. Through his help, the two staffs agreed on a process in which a committee of eight physicians would select department chairs. Four physicians from each organization would consider candidates and conduct interviews. The process required five of eight votes to elect department chairs, and it went well until the time came to choose the "big enchilada," the department of medicine chair. After a lengthy stalemate, the committee asked a respected physician to attend one of its meetings and share his views and vision on how the department of medicine should be organized and operated. He ended up being offered the position of chair, which he had not sought. Nonetheless, as the newly elected chair of Medicine, Martin Brotman, MD, supported the merger of the medical staffs because in not doing so, "you just perpetuate the problems that got you here." He successfully led the department of medicine on a campaign of "do it here" to encourage physicians to bring their business to the newly merged entity.[31]

Rolling forward two years, the leadership of the merged hospitals attempted to react to the environment of the day, believing managed care would make hospitals a commodity. The strategy announced to respond to this perceived new reality caused key physicians to leave CPMC. A significant financial challenge ensued, with the board making the decision that new leadership was required. As revenues slid significantly in the newly merged entity, costs could not be cut fast enough. Brotman, having no aspirations for a hospital executive job, was nevertheless asked to serve as CEO.

Having accepted the position, Brotman set out to create a culture of safety and accountability in the merged entity to stabilize and grow the organization. The elements of this culture included the following elements:

- *Operating under a physician-driven vision.* Brotman believes in a physician-driven organization (this does not mean that a physician must be CEO, but the vision requires the organization to have physicians in leadership and decision-making positions). Physicians are involved in all key conversations. As he puts it, "How you treat and show your respect to the physicians lets them know if physician-driven is real." In a turnaround where emphasis was placed on cost cutting, Brotman developed a growth strategy, taking no fewer than sixty initiatives to the board and medical staff. As he stated, "You can cut cost to the bone, but you can't cut into the bone."[32] He laid the foundation for behavior change with a vision and a realistic plan for growth that people could embrace.
- *Knowing your limits.* Brotman knew he was not experienced at running hospital operations, so before even accepting the CEO job, he chose his COO from the turnaround firm that was assisting CPMC at that time. Jack

Bailey served as the organization's COO for the ensuing fifteen years.

- *Maintaining honesty.* Above all else, tell the truth. If mistakes are made, such as hiring someone to a key position who is not a good fit for the organization, admit it and fix the situation quickly. In addition, in a city where unions are a strong part of the culture, CPMC leadership understands that people are free to speak and free to listen.

- *Keeping promises.* Credibility and trust are built by words *and* actions. As with any successful culture, Brotman and Bailey understand that many organizations say the right thing, but small actions demonstrate the meaning and commitment behind the words. For instance, when senior management attends medical executive committee meetings, they sit along the wall. The table is for the physicians; it is their meeting. Capital budgets are developed with deep involvement of the medical staff leadership. And in dealing with various medical staff issues, senior management does not put the board between management and the medical staff. Matters are resolved in a physician-driven format, the product of a successfully developed team culture.

    Contrast this with a merger in a southern state where one announced major objective was to implement across the system the best practices found within each organization. That "promise" soon proved to be lip service, as one executive put it, when the best practices identified within the smaller hospital were continually passed over. This trend continued until it was realized and agreed that the information technology platform at the smaller hospital was a more functional and economic investment for the system. After that, the entity began operating more like a merger than an acquisition, but the trust levels had already been compromised through broken promises.

- *Living by your principles.* "If you do not, they become fungible."[33] As Drucker states, top management needs to be sure effective behavior is actually being practiced. In his view, members of senior management need to ask themselves whether what they and the entire organization do produces the results that have been agreed upon as the necessary ones.[34] Two culture pillars uphold the vision and strategic direction of CPMC: accountability and safety. Accountability as a hallmark of this culture means that meeting agreed-upon milestones and metrics has been embedded, and a system for taking timely corrective action is equally prominent. As Brotman counsels regarding the second pillar, safety, "Don't stop listening to people, or else they'll stop talking."[35]

As mentioned in chapter 1, after CPMC stabilized its financial situation, it joined the Sutter organization and has enjoyed fifteen years as a successful merger, with key members of the senior leadership team in place through this entire period. The CEO is indeed the cornerstone for building culture in mergers.

How to Build a Successful Culture

More than one executive has acknowledged that leadership tends to overestimate its ability to make a merger work and to underestimate its ability to blend cultures. Mergers cause employees and physicians, and even senior leaders, to look inward—what will happen to me, my job, and my benefits? Will my program or department survive? What will happen to my hospital? Will I have to relocate, or face a longer drive to work? Will I even have a job?

In this chapter, we cite a number of mergers whose culture differences led to years of frustration, along with costing significant time, money, and talent. The last of Drucker's five deadly sins is *feeding problems and starving opportunities.* Drucker challenges organizations to identify their top performers and determine their assigned roles. His point is, if your organization's best people are assigned to problems, then who is taking care of the opportunities?[36] If the opportunities in mergers are left to fend for themselves, your competitors will be quite pleased.

A starting point for addressing the culture compatibility question is the *vision* for the merged entity. As the biblical proverb states, "Where there is no vision the people perish."[37] The outcome of a vision should be a transaction that makes good business sense—and importantly, makes good patient care sense. We reviewed a transaction earlier (St. Hope) in which the primary objective was to gain a significant increase in market share, which it achieved the day the deal closed. But not much of significance has happened in the years since, and in fact, market share has been lost over the years because of the internal struggle. The culture issues call into question the merit or business sense of the transaction. Remember, clean deals bring pieces and constituents together; things line up. Getting people to look up and out (rather than down and in) is the key to balancing the vision equation. This view focuses thinking and behavior toward external aims: where the customer is located and what health care needs will be provided—if not by your organization, then by another that will surely step in and provide the service.

The second step is to resolve the question of competing *values*. What are the values of your health care system or hospital? What are those of the other organization(s)? Are they compatible? Can we translate these values into a single organization in which trust can be fostered? Perhaps one way to think about values is to describe your own organization as if it were a person. Then describe the other organization the same way. If one organization is a slow-moving, risk-averse type and the other is an athlete in training for a gold medal, then bridging these two cultures will be a challenge.

Similarly, a so-called merger of equals can make it challenging to develop core values. Though numerous mergers are touted as mergers of equals, in reality, very few actually are;

furthermore, the promotion of such can lead to culture conflict. As one executive put it, "a merger of equals is a poison"[38]
when the financial, operational, and clinical metrics indicate a
situation quite different from organizational equality. Agreement on values is fundamental to building trust. Trust is built
every day, and when it is broken, it takes a long time to repair—
and sometimes it cannot be repaired.

In building trust, the leadership must create a climate in
which the truth is heard and the facts, both good and bad, are
dealt with. There is a difference between the opportunity to
have your say and the opportunity to be heard. In the research
conducted by Jim Collins, author of the book *Good to Great*, he
finds that great leaders understand this distinction and create
a culture wherein people have an opportunity to be heard and
for the truth to be known.[39] As it pertains to leaders, executive
credibility is the sum of one's expertise and the trust engendered by interactions with people that include our words, our
actions, and the degree to which we actively listen.[40]

One merger reviewed by the author involved two faith-
based organizations coming together in a unique situation in
which both parties agreed campus consolidation was in order.
But shortly after the merger was consummated, the minority
party viewed the majority party as having misrepresented its
financial strength and commitments. Despite the dominant
organization believing it had an ironclad agreement that could
not be broken, the merger ended, but not without the parties
spending several years in court as well as millions of dollars. In
short, trust could not be repaired.

In hindsight, the executive in charge of the merger for the
bigger system described this deal as "two drunks who when
sober would have never signed up for this." He stated that
the culture issues were significant, characterized by a lack of
appreciation for each other's values. Combined with ego, politics, and greed, the culture conflicts put an end to a deal that
on paper made considerable business and patient care sense. To

avoid such an outcome, successful organizations such as Bay-Care took the time to involve many people in reaching agreement about the values that would be shared among a group of religious and secular not-for-profit hospitals.[41,42]

Tenet Healthcare Corporation is another example in which shared values have helped sustain its success through ups and downs over the years. Tenet was formed in 1995 by bringing together American Medical International and National Medical Enterprise, two companies that shared a passion for being market and business development driven, that both were headquartered in California, and that both were composed of managers loyal to the company's business purposes.[43]

At CHI, its first CEO, Pat Cahill, and her team spent several months developing the core values that would be an important element in creating the CHI culture. They held 57 regional focus groups involving almost 700 participants. Each individual identified three or four essential qualities that he or she felt were important to be part of the newly merged organization going forward.

Focus groups narrowed down the proposed core values from 172 words to a half dozen. Finally, a national group of twenty-five people who had participated in earlier groups chose the four core values that have since guided the development of CHI: reverence, integrity, compassion, and excellence.[44] Getting the value component right is imperative to the success of mergers.

The third step in building a culture is to determine *what is important* and *what is not important*. As an executive or trustee, and as a member of your organization, put yourself in the other party's shoes and try to appreciate what might be important to them and what might not be so important. Given that many U.S. hospitals are components of religious ministry and outreach, the example that follows, from outside the hospital industry, illustrates the impact on an organization's culture when its leaders understand and communicate what is important and why.

Mountain Christian Church, a nondenominational church in Joppa, Maryland, has been led over the last dozen or so years by Pastor Ben Cachiaras. During this time, attendance at services has grown from several hundred to nearly 4,000 on Sunday morning, with dozens of additional activities taking place every day of the week. How does a church experiencing this kind of rapid growth, with programs that depend on volunteers for their operation, develop a culture that keeps a sense of unity and purpose among a diverse population? Its mission statement—one sentence, but unmistakably clear—is "Making disciples more and better disciples."

But perhaps the key to its success is how it goes about building its culture, as indicated by figure 4-1.[45]

We have seen mergers fail because merging the medical staffs became an obstacle. On the other hand, we have seen executives realize that merging medical staffs is "non-essential" in their markets and seen some, such as those at Alta Bates Summit, maintain separate medical staffs more than a decade after a successful merger.[46]

Why jeopardize a sound strategic deal over non-essentials? The smart leaders *know* what is important. When Holmes Regional Medical Center in Melbourne, Florida, merged with Cape Canaveral Hospital to form Health First, Mike Means, who came from Holmes to take the system CEO job, had a

Figure 4-1.   Building Culture: What Is Important for Mountain Christian Church

Unity in the essentials	A short list of statements comprising the core beliefs
Liberty in the non-essentials	Many issues that, when put under the light of the essentials, simply are not all that important in the larger strategic picture
Respect in all things	Exemplified by the church with the word *love,* and by business with the word *respect*

more formal dress code than did Larry Garrison's more informal Cape Canaveral Hospital. Garrison became the system
chief operating officer, and Means trusted Garrison to set the
dress code (mustaches are now allowed),[47] a function of the
developing culture, and demonstrated a command of what is
essential versus non-essential. Fifteen years later, these two
executives continue to serve as Health First's leaders.

Merging fund-raising organizations may be another example, with foundations in some communities having deep historical roots and being a source of pride for community leaders.
Some successfully merged entities took several years to achieve
merged fund-raising organizations. For example, Morton
Plant took two years,[48] while Health First took ten years.[49] In
another merger, the fund-raising organizations were left alone,
so that they operate outside of the merged entities. Merging
the foundations was not considered critical to the success of
these hospital mergers. In fact, Novant Health, headquartered
in Winston-Salem, North Carolina, has five foundations among
its twelve merged and acquired hospital facilities.[50]

Ascertaining what is important within your organization's
environment and culture is best considered in the preparation
of a business plan before the deal is finalized. Business plans
tend to bring to the surface hot-button issues and hidden agendas, which are important to determining the culture fit of the
organizations. Organizations that can differentiate the essentials from the non-essentials will be well positioned to establish
the business and culture fit of a transaction.

Fourth, building a culture takes *time*, perhaps more than
one would think. Many of the not-for-profit leaders interviewed for this book indicated it was anywhere from three to
six years before the new organization's sense of culture truly
had traction. Some executives indicated that it was not unrea-
sonable to think in terms of a decade before a set of new mores
and fresh storytellers could take hold in a merged organization.
This timeline is likely shorter in for-profit hospital companies,

where profit expectations drive behavior and performance in more defined time frames and heightened accountability focuses leaders on what needs to be done sooner rather than later if they expect to keep their executive positions. "Speed to value," that is, improving shareholder value, is how one executive with experience in both for-profit and not-for-profit systems characterized this priority setting when comparing the time to integrate investor-owned cultures.[51] It does not mean that one is better than the other; the two ownership models are just different.

The for-profits are more driven by financial performance and have a more singular focus in integrating cultures, while not-for-profits face a more complicated integration process, wherein financial performance is one, albeit important, consideration in the context of a broader range of mission initiatives. Communication, especially consistency in sending messages, helps accelerate the timeline.[52]

For Roger Longenderfer, MD, CEO of PinnacleHealth in Harrisburg, Pennsylvania, this means management dedicates time to building the culture. He believes in being visible as CEO and expects the same of his management team. Issues are always present to keep him at his desk, but he makes the time to get out of the office and promote the very values the culture endorses. He personally leads all employee orientations to speak to the issues of mission and values. Furthermore, he tells employees to call or e-mail him if they do not see his management team regularly.[53]

Another executive agrees about the importance of visibility, but goes further by saying that making rounds needs to be purposeful. Visibility is more than just walking around and waving; it means taking time to ask questions, *listen*, and let people know by words and actions that you care.[54] These efforts contribute to accelerating the timeline to building culture.

Finally, our interviews and observations indicated the cornerstone of the culture fit and success of a merged organization was the selection of the CEO. Paul Wiles, CEO of Novant Health, confirmed his own view of this, indicating that culture differences were his most significant challenge in pulling together the mid-1990s merger between hospitals located in Winston-Salem and Charlotte, about seventy miles apart. He came to appreciate and agree with something that he had heard from someone else, that, indeed, "culture is the shadow of the CEO."[55]

Handling the culture issues in a merger is significantly more difficult than handling an outright acquisition. As one executive from a large system noted, in acquisitions it is their way or the highway; the acquiring entity removes the local board, holds the right to replace management, and gives management about one year to "get it"—they best learn how to deal with the way the bigger organization conducts its business affairs.

Mergers' success hinges on the organizations' ability to meet that challenge of changing behavior from the inward, protectionist mode (What is going to happen to me?) to looking up and out and embracing the challenge of a new vision for delivering health care services. As best-selling author Thomas Friedman put it, "You want constantly to acquire new skills, knowledge, and expertise that enable you constantly to be able to create value."[56] This advice pertains to both organizations and individuals. Those organizations in which people are included in learning and crafting the change, rather then being mandated to make the change, fair better at successful implementation of the desired result.

The merged entity's new CEO must be able to generate the climate that engenders the behavior change to achieve the results required to make the merger successful. Figure 4-2 summarizes the steps to building a corporate culture in a merged health system.

The challenge for executives and board members is to take a realistic look at the culture and business issues facing a prospective merged organization and determine whether "their" executive is really the right fit for the CEO role of the merged entity or the "right" call is to go in a different direction. In chapter 5, we delve into the selection process.

Figure 4-2.   Building a Merged Health System Corporate Culture

Vision	A compelling business and clinical case is made for the merger.
Values	Core beliefs that engender trust are identified.
Essentials versus non-essentials	The strategic business plan spells out what is important and how/when it will be accomplished.
Time	Management and board live and communicate the vision and values and monitor milestones/ metrics and commitment.
CEO	The chief executive rallies stakeholders, translates vision into practice, and transfers practice into accountability.

References

1. Terrence E. Deal and Allan A. Kennedy, *Corporate Cultures: The Rites and Rituals of Corporate Life* (Reading, MA: Addison-Wesley, 1982), 4.
2. *Hospitals & Health Networks*, "America's Top 100 Integrated Systems," *Hospitals and Health Networks* 72, no. 6 (1998): 38–39.
3. Bernard (Bernie) L. Brown, CEO PROMINA Health System (retired), interview with author, Atlanta, July 16, 2009.
4. Bonnie Phipps, CEO, St. Agnes Hospital, Baltimore, and former CEO, PROMINA Health System, interview with author, Baltimore, July 1, 2009.
5. Brown interview.
6. Brown interview.
7. Robert Stanek, CEO, Catholic Health East (retired), interview with author, Newtown Square, Pennsylvania, July 15, 2009.
8. Deal and Kennedy, *Corporate Cultures*, 13–15.
9. Peter F. Drucker, *Managing for the Future: The 1990s and Beyond* (New York: Truman Talley Books/Dutton, 1992), 191.
10. Mike Sellards, CEO, St. Mary's Hospital and Palatine Health System, interview with author, Huntington, West Virginia, July 9, 2009.
11. J. Thomas Jones, CEO, West Virginia United Health System, interview with author, Fairmont, West Virginia, July 10, 2009.
12. Mike Perry, former trustee and board chair, Genesis Hospital System, interview with author, Huntington, West Virginia, July 9, 2009.

13. Warren Kirk, CEO, and Robert Petrina, chief financial officer, Alta Bates Summit Medical Center, interview with author, Oakland, California, July 22, 2009.
14. Michael Means, CEO, and Larry Garrison, COO, Health First, interview with author, Rockledge, Florida, June 24, 2009.
15. Ronald R. Aldrich, former CEO, Franciscan Health System, interview with author, Hope, Idaho, June 29, 2009.
16. Jaan Sidorov, "Case Study of a Failed Merger of Hospital Systems," *Managed Care* 12, no. 11 (2003): 56–60.
17. Ibid.
18. Ibid.
19. Peter F. Drucker, *Managing in a Time of Great Change* (New York: Truman Talley Books/Dutton, 1995), 48.
20. Peggy Noonan, "Keep Robert Gates," *Wall Street Journal,* November 22, 2008: A15.
21. Reynold Jennings, former COO, Tenet Healthcare Corporation, interview with author, October 27, 2009.
22. *Life Application Bible, New International Version* (Wheaton, IL: Tyndale, 1991), James 2:17, p. 2248.
23. Terrence O'Rourke, MD, chief clinical officer, Trinity Health System, interview with author, Novi, Michigan, August 12, 2009.
24. Joseph R. Swedish, president and CEO, Trinity Health System, interview with author, Novi, Michigan, November 6, 2009.
25. Pat Shehorn, CEO, Westlake Hospital and West Suburban Medical Center, interview with author, Chicago, August 19, 2009.
26. Drucker, *Managing for the Future*, 192.
27. Ibid., 193–194.
28. Frank Murphy, former CEO, Morton Plant and Morton Plant Mease Health, and CEO (retired), BayCare Health System, interview with author, St. Petersburg, Florida, August 10, 2009.
29. Ibid.
30. Craig Brethauer, vice president, Human Resources, BayCare Health System, interview with author, St. Petersburg, Florida, August 10, 2009.
31. Martin Brotman, MD, CEO, California Pacific Medical Center, interview with author, San Francisco, July 22, 2009.
32. Ibid.
33. Ibid.
34. Drucker, *Managing for the Future*, 194–195.
35. Martin Brotman, MD, CEO, and Jack Bailey, COO, California Pacific Medical Center, interview with author, San Francisco, July 22, 2009.
36. Drucker, *Managing in a Time of Great Change*, 49.

37. Frank Charles Thompson, *The New Chain-Reference Bible* (Indiana-polis: B.B. Kirkbride Bible Co., 1964), 630.
38. Paul Wiles, CEO, Novant Health, interview with author, Winston-Salem, North Carolina, February 18, 2010.
39. Jim Collins, *Good to Great: Why Some Companies Make the Leap . . . and Others Don't* (New York: HarperCollins, 2001), 74.
40. Mary Nash, PhD, RN, chief nurse executive and associate vice president for health sciences, Ohio State Health System, interview with author, Columbus, Ohio, December 1, 2009.
41. Murphy interview.
42. Phillip K. Beauchamp, CEO (retired) Morton Plant Mease Health, interview with author, Dunedin, Florida, June 26, 2009.
43. Jennings interview.
44. Patricia A. Cahill and Maryanna Coyle, *Catholic Health Initiatives, a Spirit of Innovation, a Legacy of Care, the Early Years* (Denver: Catholic Health Initiatives, 2006), 144–145.
45. Mountain Christian Church, new member class orientation manual, p.5.
46. Kirk interview.
47. Means interview.
48. Beauchamp interview.
49. Means interview.
50. Wiles interview.
51. Swedish interview.
52. Robert Troy, human resources consultant, interview with author, Katonah, New York, July 2–3, 2009.
53. Roger Longenderfer, MD, president and CEO, PinnacleHealth System, interview with author, Harrisburg, Pennsylvania, August 3, 2009.
54. Nash interview.
55. Wiles interview.
56. Thomas L. Friedman, *The World Is Flat: A Brief History of the Twenty-First Century* (New York: Farrar, Straus and Giroux, 2005), 239.

5

Choosing the CEO, Board, and Management Team

Deal breakers—every transaction has them. Deal breakers often have little to do with the core business merits of the transaction and more to do with perceptions about who or what it will take to get the deal done and make the transaction successful. They usually revolve around the following critical points:

1. Who will be the chief executive officer (CEO)?
2. Who will comprise the initial board, and who will be the first board chair?
3. Who will comprise the initial senior management team?

Hospital deals that otherwise make sound business sense and potentially provide significant community benefit can be called off because the proposed answers to these questions are not satisfactory to one of the parties. In fact, a few executives interviewed were aware of a recently proposed merger that would have been a headliner, but neither CEO would agree to work for the other as chief executive of the merged entity, thus the deal fell apart. As one health system executive expressed, "90% of mergers are based on personalities."[1]

In this chapter we look at several cases that provide lessons in addressing these questions.

Choosing the Chief Executive Officer

A number of factors are involved in selecting the CEO for a merged health care entity. Some of the more subtle, albeit important, variables are discussed in the following scenarios.

Knowing One's Own Strengths and Limits

One day in February 1997, Bill Kerr was named CEO of the newly formed merger of the University of California, San Francisco and Stanford health care organizations. Later that evening, Kerr changed his mind about accepting the CEO position. He called key leaders to inform them of his reasons.

After nearly two years of work bringing together these two renowned academic medical centers, Kerr, then CEO of University of California, San Francisco Medical Center (UCSF), recalls that the process for choosing a CEO seemed to go quickly. The new board for UCSF Stanford Health Care was appointed in January 1997. A committee interviewed the leaders from each side, Kerr from UCSF and Peter Van Etten from Stanford. Kerr recalls the press waiting outside the room to interview the successful candidate. After his appointment, he decided he could better serve the organization as chief operating officer (COO) of the merged entity, not the organizational front man with its own demands of a CEO. He truly felt Van Etten would be more appropriate in the CEO role, and he as the COO.

Kerr also criticized himself for not flagging the committee and slowing down the process of choosing the first CEO of the merged enterprise. He offered to step aside so that Van Etten could choose his own COO, but Van Etten asked Kerr to stay on as executive vice president and chief operating officer, the number two executive. Kerr believes that Van Etten and he worked well together in their respective roles in the two short years the merger lasted.[2]

Kerr is known nationally as the successful and long-tenured CEO of UCSF. However, in a merger that combined two strong academic medical centers, Kerr felt his strength—what he enjoyed most, and what would be best for the new organization—was to serve in the number two role of the combined organization.

Few successful executives can critique their own strength and suppress their ego and professional standing to do what is truly best for the organization, the stakeholders, and the community. Many executives say they want to do the "right thing," but not many willingly withdraw before, let alone after, the selection is announced. To remove himself from such an illustrious and high-salaried position, or for that matter from almost any hospital CEO role, was a true reflection of Kerr's character, confidence, class, and humility.

Knowing one's strengths, as well as limits, serves executives and merged organizations well. Boards need to thoughtfully consider executive fit in merged organizations and are wise to follow the mantra of former President Ronald Reagan, "Trust but verify," when internal executives nominate themselves for senior roles.

When Newness Is a Disadvantage—or an Advantage

Certainly, merger opportunities have come to an end because on one side or the other a new chief executive was recently hired or joined an organization in the midst of the deliberation. What new CEO wants to jeopardize a new position he or she just recently started? Few would do it. One merger in the mid-1990s was announced when the definitive agreement was signed (think of being at the altar, with only the "I do" remaining to be said), but the arrival of a new CEO on one side of the transaction soon brought the deal to an end before it could be finalized.

But newness does not always have to be a disadvantage. When Morton Plant and Mease Health Care were in discussions about a merger, Morton Plant, the larger organization, insisted its executive, Frank Murphy, be named the CEO of the merged enterprise—it was a deal breaker. Murphy was fairly new to his position as CEO, having taken over for a long-tenured executive who had retired.

On the Mease Health Care side, Phil Beauchamp was also new to his position. Considering the dynamics taking place in the market, Beauchamp was attempting, along with his board, to make critical strategic decisions for his organization. Given his many years of chief executive experience, he did not feel threatened about making a decision for his organization that might not be in his own best interest professionally. Despite the competitiveness of the two organizations, Beauchamp felt neither he nor Murphy had any history of hardened feelings from past actions and decisions; on the other hand, their respective newness helped facilitate a rational dialogue between the two organizations.[3] As described in chapter 4, when Murphy was selected as CEO, he, being sensitive to Beauchamp's position, created an "office of the president." He moved his office to Beauchamp's location and promised the two would work together.[4] Though Murphy was clearly the CEO, he won Beauchamp's trust, and the two worked closely together from the merger's inception in 1994 until Murphy's retirement in 2004. When Morton Plant Mease became part of an even larger organization in 1996, BayCare Health System, Beauchamp took over Murphy's former position as president and CEO of Morton Plant Mease. Trust between two key (and formerly competing) executives and a strong commitment to make the transaction work fostered a successful merger of these organizations. One former operations executive credits these two executives for making this merger work by not letting their egos get in the way. As he reflected, they never put the board in the middle; they worked well together to resolve organizational challenges and issues.[5]

Going Outside for the CEO

There is no rule of thumb to guide an organization as to whether to go outside the organization or stay inside in the search for a merged organization's new CEO. However, there is this rule: Get it right, and the business purpose and culture have a good chance of success; get it wrong, and the merger will be compromised.

In the 1990s, when three health care systems representing religious congregations were forming what would become a dynamic national transaction known as Catholic Health Initiatives (CHI), one of the more sensitive issues was whether any of the three chief executive officers should be considered for the CEO position of the merged entity.

The forming system's steering council reflected on the skills needed to manage the new organization and sought a leader whose profile and style stretched the traditional model. This executive would bring the following traits:

- Collaboration skills
- Strong team-building skills
- Communication skills, as one who could build consensus and participation
- Vision, as one who would be enthusiastic about the mission and vision of Catholic health care
- Health care strategy and oversight competency
- Recognition and appreciation of the leadership contribution of women religious to the ministry who themselves possessed a deep sense of ministry[6]

Ron Aldrich, former CEO of one of the founding organizations, the Franciscan Health System, located outside of Philadelphia, recalls his own struggle over who would be best suited for the CEO position of the proposed new and very large national Catholic hospital system. He believed that the first CEO needed to be Roman Catholic, which effectively removed him from consideration, assuming inside candidates were to be considered. Aldrich described reaching this conclusion as being "very freeing." He could then give his best advice without any self-conflict.[7] Aldrich makes a significant point for health system boards and sponsors to consider: It is difficult for sitting executives to make objective decisions when they are campaigning for a job in the proposed merged entity. All three CEOs of the founding health systems were successful executives; however, they accepted the decision of the forming system's steering council to look for an external candidate for the CEO position.[8] Three external candidates were interviewed for the position.[9] Patricia Cahill was chosen as the first CEO of CHI, a position she held from its inception in 1996 until her retirement in 2003. None of the three founding chief executives took positions in the merged entity.

In a separate merger case, the former CEO of a Catholic-Protestant merger, which has struggled for years to achieve true merger benefits, observed—with the benefit of five years of hindsight—that perhaps it would have been best for the board to have sought a CEO from outside the organization rather than choosing the other party's CEO. A new independent leader, rather than an executive chosen from one of the founding entities, might have provided a better basis by which to bring the merger to a successfully functioning enterprise.

When the CEO's Career Timeline Affects Mergers

Age matters. A CEO's career timeline can influence his or her enthusiasm and ability to endorse a potential merger. Chief executives and others in senior management naturally are concerned about the impact of a proposed merger on their own career. Regardless of sound rationale for a transaction, a merger could mean diminishment in title and responsibility or, worse, the loss of a job, likely meaning uprooting family in the search for a new executive position.

Thus, age can be an impediment. Whether CEOs are a few years from retirement or in the prime of their career, they are in a position to influence their boards' view on the merits of a proposed merger. Making decisions that could disrupt a "secure" job and lifestyle has ended any number of merger prospects. The risk and possible changes for such executives are not viewed as more rewarding than the status quo. Just as there are only so many head coaching jobs in sports, there are only so many CEO jobs in health care. As mentioned in chapter 4 in the discussion on culture, a proposed change has to be better than the current status quo for most professionals to embrace it. Achieving this goal is easier said than done under the time constraints and stress brought about by merger opportunities.

Age, however, can also be an advantage. Ron Aldrich observed that the sister-leaders of the three founding congregations of CHI, plus the two sister-CEOs of Sisters of Charity (Cincinnati, Ohio) and Catholic Health Corporation (Omaha, Nebraska), were all women in the final years of their career or appointment. He felt this allowed them to be more future oriented and gave them the ability to be courageous.[10] As one system merger and acquisition executive put it, "Sometimes age makes it easier, but it is a case-by-case situation."[11]

The factors of age and career plans can, thankfully, be trumped by the presence of executives who see the big picture and/or have respect for the executive(s) sitting on the other side of the negotiating table. When Larry Garrison, former CEO of Cape Canaveral Hospital, and Mike Means, CEO of the larger Holmes Regional Medical Center, and their respective boards were negotiating their merger in the mid-1990s, Garrison felt all along that Means would be the right person for the CEO position, even though both were executives with many career years ahead of them. Garrison knew his hospital needed a capital partner and would have to merge with another organization.[12] He understood the big picture. In addition, these two executives shared a mutual respect despite the competition for patients. The merger consummated in 1994, and Means and Garrison continue to hold the CEO and COO positions, respectively, at Health First sixteen years post-merger.

Here we offer a brief word about co–chief executive officers: They do not work, as indicated by examples in previous chapters. One CEO recalled an experience he had with a co-CEO role. He described it as the worst eighteen months of his life. When the merger agreement finally called for the selection of a singular CEO, he was chosen; however, the other co-CEO was not pleased with this choice and thereafter went about the process of breaking up the merger, in which he was in fact successful.

Figure 5-1 lists the factors that affect CEO selection in merged organizations.

Choosing the New Board

In a merger, one of the more sensitive issues is deciding the composition of the new system's board. Should the new board be composed of a significant number of new members? Or should it be a representative body reflecting the ownership structure? Just as with the decision whether to seek a CEO from inside the organization or outside, there is no cookie-cutter approach to determining the members of the new board. That said, getting it right is imperative to a successful merger; getting it wrong can be costly and even lead to failure.

Figure 5-1.   Factors Affecting CEO Selection in Mergers

Organization's complexity and size	
CEO's:	Experience
	Age
	Newness to organization
	Values compared with legacy culture's
	Grasp of mission and vision: ability to articulate, get others to embrace them
	Team-building expertise
	Communication skills: internal and external

Let us look at several cases to glean what works and what does not work in the new board selection process.

Representative Boards

Centura Health of Denver was formed in 1996 from a joint venture of Catholic Health Initiatives and Adventist Health System. Its first board chair, Terrence O'Rourke, MD, noted the system board was composed of the chairs of all the hospital boards. As such, the board was representative, with each member looking out for his or her own entity and harboring little appreciation of the role and function of a system board. The initial years of the merger were marked by a financial crisis, which provided a platform for restructuring the board.[13] A change in board structure and new management were catalysts for Centura's ensuing success.

In another example, a Midwest system CEO spoke about the merger of his organization with another organization. From a financial and business perspective the merger was very successful, removing an average of $50 million in costs per year in the first five years. The new board was composed of 50 percent membership from each merging party, reflecting the equal ownership structure. However, the two organizations brought very different cultures to the deal, and the differences started in the boardroom. Each side had different views of how a board should conduct business, including conflicting philosophies on dealing with board-vendor relationships. Board meetings during this time were contentious. Finally, after five frustrating years, both parties acknowledged that someone needed to take control and buy the other party out of the merger. This CEO's system decided to buy out the other party and take full control. Not long thereafter, a physician group sought to build a new, competing hospital, later enlisting another large system to assist it in achieving the goal. As this system CEO noted, a merger that should have been good for the broader community failed, and if that were not enough, a new competitor emerged out of it. The leadership and cultural failures in the boardroom were costly in more ways than one.

In yet another example, PROMINA Health was voted the number one integrated delivery system in the United States in 1998. However, the system board structure, consisting of one board member from each organization and the respective CEOs, fostered a representative environment rather than a system board. As noted in chapter 4, the perceived lack of value as a system led to its demise a few years after receiving its high-profile accolade.[14]

Bringing merged boards together with an agreement to turn the board over within a specified timeline is one way to prevent representative boards from staying in place. For instance, when Morton Plant and Mease came together, the chairman of Morton Plant remembers calling a meeting with the chairman of Mease and the two CEOs to work out the board issue, among other items to be addressed. On the board issue, agreement was reached to bring all twenty-two members from both boards forward to the merged entity, but a timetable was put in place to pare the board down to fifteen members over three years. After a few years, new members coming in had no legacy perspectives but were instead focused on the new entity known as Morton Plant Mease.

The former board chairman remarked that a key element in making this process work was the fact that both boards had term limits, which facilitated a transition to a board singularly focused on the merged entity. Furthermore, members of both boards were committed to making the merger work and supported the transition plan.[15]

Sponsor Conflicts

Because so many U.S. hospitals were founded on and continue to be associated with religious organizations, we note their influence on mergers, even though they may delegate some or even substantial powers to health system boards that focus on the hospital ministry.

One executive related the story of a new faith-based system being formed in the Midwest in the 1990s. This executive was interviewed as an outside candidate for the first CEO position of the new system and was selected. A short time later, he was informed that a sister who was not picked for the CEO role would be the full-time board chair and would be located in the executive suite. The CEO, upon learning that news, respectfully declined to take the position. The system disbanded within a couple of years.[16]

In another example, a CEO recalled his efforts to merge his organization with another system that would have provided a powerful faith-based entity in a wider geographic market. His organization, the larger of the two, was run by a health system board with substantial authority, while in the other system the sponsors, rather than the health system board, held all the power. The smaller system demanded a continuance of its philosophy and history of equal sponsorship, which was a deal breaker for the larger system. The merger discussions never got beyond the sponsor conflicts, and the larger organization took a pass on an otherwise apparently good business deal for each of the sponsor's hospitals.

In yet another case, a recent effort to merge two large organizations failed when, at one key meeting, the sponsor of one organization failed to show up. That sponsor already had a reputation for arrogance. The excuse for not making the meeting was viewed as weak and the absence an act of disrespect, and this reaction led to the termination of what would have been a headline merger.

One final case of note, the Daughters of Charity of the Province of the West merged with Catholic Healthcare West (CHW) in 1995. In 2001, this system pulled out of CHW, in part because of the differences in sponsor role, with the sisters of the Daughters of Charity of the Province of the West believing in a more hands-on approach than was practiced by the entity. Robert Issai, current president and CEO of the Daughters of Charity Health System, believes co-sponsorships are a challenge to make work, given inherent conflicts stemming from the history and heritage of the respective congregations. Furthermore, he feels that mergers of Catholic hospitals with non-Catholic hospitals become "Catholic lite," not a very compelling case for the mission in his view.[17]

First Board Chair

Just as the first CEO sets the critical cultural and operational tone for a merged organization, the first board chair reflects the governance and community attitude of the merged enterprise. If the first board chair continues to represent his or her legacy hospital or system, a tone and culture of dysfunction will be established that the rest of the members will likely follow. If, however, the first board chair reflects the newly merged organization and holds the board and management accountable for the strategic direction and operational and financial performance of the merged organization, the governance is off to an excellent start.

One prospective merger, despite its strategic merits, fell apart at least in part over the selection of the first board chair. While the larger organization insisted that its CEO be the first chief executive of the merged entity (a deal killer), the smaller organization countered that its board chair be the first chair of the merged organization. Right or wrong, the larger organization viewed the recommended board chair as a protectionist, someone who could not bring stakeholders together on behalf of the larger health system. The merger discussions came to a halt.

An executive from a for-profit company observed that his company's ability to acquire two hospitals from a failed not-for-profit hospital merger stemmed from a lack of leadership at the board level to drive the strategic change needed to make the merger successful.

The selection of the first board chair is much more than a negotiating position for the power seats. If the organizations get this decision wrong, as we have seen in several cases, the merger will be compromised in its intention to reach its potential or even fail. Selecting a first board chair who can bring together stakeholders to focus on a new organization with a new vision and strategic direction is a critical element in the success of a merger. Subsequent board chairs then have a model and mentor to follow that should serve the organization well in the ensuing years.

Ensuring Effective Governance

A predictor of success of any organization is the effectiveness of its governance. Almost any distressed organization's problems can be traced back to ineffective governance.

Just look at the troubles of the companies whose performance headlined the recent economic crisis in the United States, and one cannot help but ask, What was the governing body doing in the months and years leading to the collapse of these companies? For distressed hospitals and health systems, questions about organizational performance need to be asked first in the boardroom, where such trouble usually begins or perpetuates.

Some mergers bring together all the board members of both organizations and commence the merger with a large board, perhaps paring it down over time, such as we have seen at Morton Plant Mease. The larger the size, the more time-consuming it is to conduct business.

Other organizations attempt to choose a certain number of members from each of the merged entities to form the new board. Size is certainly a consideration, but more importantly, the focus must be on governance of the new combined entity: future oriented, not anchored in representing the previous legacy organizations.

When the Daughters of Charity in St. Louis, Missouri, and the Sisters of St. Joseph, in Michigan, merged in 1999 to form Ascension Health System, an entirely new board was formed of members having no previous association with the founding entities.[18] This approach focused governance and organizational performance on the new entity and its future.

When California Health System (CHS) merged with Sutter Health, Sutter agreed to a board composition of 50 percent from each side; however, CHS was formerly a federation and as such had to give up substantial autonomy in the merger to focus on the newly combined organization.[19]

Doug Hawthorne, CEO of fourteen-hospital Texas Health Resources, notes that when the merger of Presbyterian and Harris hospitals in the Dallas–Fort Worth area was put together in the 1990s, emphasis was placed on forging the new system, not representing the past. After three years, the board, consisting of eighteen members, became self-perpetuating, whereby new board members are elected by existing board members. A sponsor board remains in place to hold management accountable to adhere to mission, and local boards remain in place in all fourteen hospitals.[20]

When CHI was formed in 1996, twelve board members were chosen. The board was composed of three members from each of the three founding organizations and three outsiders. The first CEO, Pat Cahill, began her job with the new board already in place. She reflects that she never worked with such a breadth and depth of talent. The board members never once represented their legacy organizations; they had an amazing ability to let go of the past. They were singularly focused on the new organization and rolled up their sleeves to take on whatever challenge needed to be met to make the mission and merger successful.[21]

Whether or not local boards remain in place at member hospitals is a question of organizational philosophy, availability of talent, or local or state regulation. Don Lorack viewed local board members as ambassadors of the system, worth the extra work and meeting time, when he ran Hillcrest Health System in Tulsa, Oklahoma.[22] Robert Stanek, former CEO of Catholic Health East (CHE), views the local board as very important, a key to the "relational culture" that constitutes CHE and a reminder that "health care is local."[23]

However, the key is the board formed at the system level, as it will set the policies and the business culture for all components of the merged organization. Health care systems and their board members will be under increasing pressure to justify future investments in technology, equipment, and buildings, along with the overall cost of providing care versus the outcomes of care. A skill-set matrix for the board should be developed, reviewed, and updated annually. Emphasis should be placed on nominating members whose skills can help the organization successfully meet its mission and its challenges. In addition, specific consideration needs to be given to selecting individuals who have the time to carry out the fiduciary responsibilities required in accepting a board position.

The board size must reflect the ability to move business at prudent speed in an environment where competitors will develop strategies to take market share; changes in technology and regulation will require deeper knowledge, operational flexibility, and timely decision making. Figure 5-2 summarizes the key considerations in selecting a board for the newly merged entity.

Figure 5-2.   New Board Selection Considerations

Purpose	Fiduciary Responsibility for New Entity
Future orientation	Focus to achieve merger objectives (not represent legacy organization)
Composition	Skill-set matrix to bring required talent to boardroom
Size	Ability to grasp issues and respond quickly (12–18 members)
Term limits	Attention to skill-set matrix and market changes that require new blood
First board chair	Promotion of oneness of new organization, mentor to new board
Accountability	Establishment and monitoring of standards for governance performance

Choosing the Initial Senior Management Team

Another sensitive issue that affects mergers and, at times, even determines whether they go forward is the selection of the senior management team, a critical factor to merger success. The positions in the senior team sometimes become negotiating points in a merger. For instance, in the merger of UCSF with Stanford Health, the fact that the first CEO came from Stanford meant, according to the terms of the negotiations, that the first chief medical officer would come from UCSF.[24]

In some merger discussions, CEOs or boards make promises to their key senior leaders that the leaders' jobs will be secure or perhaps offer them "stay" bonuses or make other compensation arrangements during these periods of uncertainty. Caution should be exercised by CEOs and boards in these matters. Merger discussions take place in a period of high anxiety not just for senior leaders but also for many others potentially affected by the contemplated change, especially employees.

However, as it pertains to senior management, the manner in which those executives handle their responsibilities in this uncertain period can be an excellent indicator of who will be a good senior leader in a merged, more complex organization. Before a CEO or board makes promises or payments to C-suite executives, they might want to consider using this period to judge the performance of the potential leaders against the backdrop of change and uncertainty. It could prove very telling and make the selection of the new senior team leaders easier. One CEO, whose organization went through a successful merger in the late 1990s, is currently in merger negotiations with another regional health system. The CEO notes that the senior leaders who viewed the merger of ten years ago as an opportunity and welcomed that change are now entrenched executives. In the current negotiations of a new merger with its uncertainties, some of these same executives are resistant to the merger, asking, Why pursue this merger? believing operations are going well. As this CEO notes, their reaction will make it easier for him and the other organization's leader to choose who stays as members of the senior management when the deal closes.

The fact is, in choosing a new senior management team, some very capable people will lose their job. Only so many senior positions are available, and attempting to placate personalities rather than dealing with the hard issues will only compromise the merger efficiencies and the new organization's effectiveness.

Sometimes organizations attempt to circumvent the difficult issue of choosing one executive over another by naming co-executives. Most organizations in other industries would never consider having two chief financial officers, for example, but somehow in health care mergers, boards at times contemplate appointing co–executive officers, co–operating officers, co–nursing officers, or co–medical officers. Co-anything in senior management does not work in the long run. One health care executive admits that his consultant's advice to not have co–chief nursing officers was indeed correct, a conclusion he and his team reached after trying to manage the situation for ten years. Another executive, whose career experience has included roles as chief nursing officer, chief operating officer, and chief executive officer and who has traveled the United States as a nurse magnet program appraiser, observed she has never seen co–senior management roles work, nor leadership by committee.[25]

Perhaps one way to remove the temptation of making senior positions a pawn in negotiations is to think about the skills that will be needed to manage a more complex organization in a health care market that is becoming increasingly competitive. Just as a merger is a good time for a board to select members with skills that contribute to carrying out its mission, it is also a good time for the chief executive(s) to step back and evaluate the types of skills required to effectively manage in the next decade or two.

Pat Cahill notes that in selecting her initial senior management team for CHI she did not concern herself with achieving representation from the three founding systems, but focused on getting the best people with the required skill sets to serve the mission and purpose of the newly merged organization. She believed then, and believes five years after retirement, that she had the best senior management team in the United States. Cahill further believes the commitment of this initial senior management team was evident when, during a three-year period of financial challenges, no incentive compensation was awarded and every executive stayed.[26]

Doug Hawthorne, CEO of Texas Health Resources, counsels to select the senior management team quickly: "Don't let it drag on." He believes the new team should be in place within sixty to ninety days.[27] Frank Murphy, former CEO of nine-hospital BayCare Health System, put his management team together in sixty days, reducing the number of vice presidents, as described in chapter 4, from fifty-two in the legacy hospitals to twenty-three in the merged enterprise.[28]

The selection of the chief nursing officer (CNO) demands a certain sensitivity and skill set. Nurses are especially conscious of the reputation of their hospitals because they are often judged by the public, their patients, and physicians. Mergers that may appear organizationally to be more or less equal do not see that quality reflected at the nursing unit level. From the nurses' view, someone wins, and someone loses. It is important that senior leaders recognize this perception and that the CNO address it. Nurses will be concerned over which hospital's reputation will prevail, which nursing model of care will continue, which hospital will need to change or cease to exist. Sometimes how support staff are used in delivering nursing care (as in the use of licensed practical nurses and nurse aides) is a function of recruitment availability in a local market, and such matters tend to get minimized in the big picture of merger strategy and tactics. In mergers, nursing styles change, policies are reformulated, and work standards are redrafted. Some nurses will lose shift or hour preference or perhaps lose their job. Change is difficult to embrace for nursing staff, as with management, unless they understand and believe that change will be better than the status quo.[29,30]

Physicians and nurses are the heart of a hospital's patient care reputation. Just as particular sensitivity must be placed on seeking an effective leader for the role of the CNO, the same can be said for the selection of the system chief medical officer. This is not meant to take away from the importance of other senior leaders, such as operations and finance officers who are clearly in critically important positions to direct resources and lead change, but the embodiment of a hospital's reputation lies in the real or perceived competence of its nurses and physicians.

Figure 5-3 summarizes the steps in choosing the senior management team for the merged organization.

Often some compromise takes place in choosing candidates for senior leadership positions, as the manner in which the organizations are blended becomes important to reflect a partnership approach rather than a takeover approach (as might be the case in an acquisition). Some good executives will lose their job; however, good executives find another job. The challenge for a merged organization's CEO and board is to fill the senior roles with executives who possess the skills required to effectively compete and embrace the vision and strategic

Figure 5-3.   Selecting the Senior Management Team

- Observe incumbents' pre-merger handling of uncertainty
- Decide on stay bonus/severance packages
- Determine skills needed for each senior position to manage a larger organization
- Review merits of selecting from in-house versus going outside
- Accountability: make hard decisions; no co–senior executives
- Finalize decision within first quarter post-closing

direction and whose values reflect the culture and behavior changes required to carry out the mission. Executives need to determine what it will take for their organizations to still be operating in the year 2020.

References

1. Michael Rowan, COO, Catholic Health Initiatives, interview with author, Denver, October 26, 2009.
2. William J. (Bill) Kerr, former CEO, University of California, San Francisco and former, COO, UCSF Stanford Health Care, interview with author, San Francisco, September 22, 2009.
3. Philip K. Beauchamp, former CEO, Morton Plant Mease Health, interview with author, Dunedin, Florida, June 26, 2009.
4. Frank Murphy, former CEO, BayCare Health System, and former CEO, Morton Plant Mease Health, interview with author, St. Petersburg, Florida, August 10, 2009.
5. James Pfeiffer, CEO, Self Regional Medical Center, interview with author, Greenwood, South Carolina, November 4, 2009.
6. Patricia A. Cahill and Maryanna Coyle, *Catholic Health Initiatives, a Spirit of Innovation, a Legacy of Care, the Early Years* (Denver: Catholic Health Initiatives, 2006), 91.
7. Ronald R. Aldrich, former CEO, Franciscan Health System, interview with author, Hope, Idaho, June 29, 2009.
8. Cahill and Coyle, *Catholic Health Initiatives*, 91.
9. Cahill and Coyle, *Catholic Health Initiatives*, 92.
10. Aldrich interview.
11. John Shea, vice president, Business Development, and vice president, Sponsorship, Bon Secours Health System, interview with author, Marriottsville, Maryland, July 7, 2009.
12. Michael Means, CEO, and Larry Garrison, COO, Health First, interview with author, Rockledge, Florida, June 24, 2009.
13. Terrence O'Rourke, MD, chief medical officer, Trinity Health, and former board chair, Centura Health, interview with author, Novi, Michigan, August 12, 2009.
14. Bernard L. (Bernie) Brown, CEO (retired), PROMINA Health, interview with author, Atlanta, July 16, 2009.
15. Alan Bomstein, former chairman of the board, Morton Plant and Morton Plant Mease Health, interview with author, Clearwater, Florida, November 2, 2009.
16. William Foley, CEO, Cook County Health and Hospital System, interview with author, Chicago, August 19, 2009.

17. Robert Issai, CEO, Daughters of Charity Health System, interview with author, Los Altos Hills, California, July 21, 2009.
18. Doug French, former CEO, Ascension Health, interview with author, St. Louis, Missouri, October 14, 2009.
19. Patrick Fry, CEO, Sutter Health, interview with author, Sacramento, California, July 20, 2009.
20. Douglas D. Hawthorne, CEO, Texas Health Resources, interview with author, Arlington, Texas, September 21, 2009.
21. Patricia A. Cahill, Esq., CEO (retired), Catholic Health Initiatives, interview with author, West Barnstable, Massachusetts, November 10, 2009.
22. Don Lorack, former CEO, Hillcrest Medical Center, interview with author, Orange County, California, July 17, 2009.
23. Robert Stanek, CEO, Catholic Health East (retired), interview with author, Newtown Square, Pennsylvania, July 15, 2009.
24. Kerr interview.
25. Mary Nash, PhD, RN, chief nurse executive and associate vice president for health sciences, Ohio State Health System, interview with author, Columbus, Ohio, December 1, 2009.
26. Cahill interview.
27. Hawthorne interview.
28. Murphy interview.
29. Peg Price, RN, principal, Insight Health Partners, interview with author, St. Petersburg, Florida, August 9, 2009.
30. Linda Kenwood, RN, consultant, e-mail interview with author, August 3, 2009.

6

Merger Outcomes: Good for the Patients and the Community?

In 1996, Harrisburg Hospital and Polyclinic Hospital, located in Harrisburg, Pennsylvania, merged to become PinnacleHealth. The cost savings benefiting the community were documented for the first five years, pursuant to an agreement with the commonwealth's attorney general. One of the key principles of the merger was to maintain acute care services at all campuses,[1] a typical agreement reached in many mergers. Two years later, a third hospital came into the Pinnacle system, primarily to resolve its own financial distress.

When the time came to deal with the always difficult issue of clinical consolidation, it became clear to the management and board of the system that the best option to achieve high-quality patient care, efficiency, and cost control was "real consolidation." Roger Longenderfer, MD, chief executive officer (CEO) of PinnacleHealth (and its former chief medical officer), remembers the sense of the board being, "Why merge if we can't consolidate." So the board made the difficult decision to put aside a key principle established going into the merger and agreed to consolidate services because that action would better serve the patients and the community. Today the Polyclinic campus is primarily an outpatient health care campus. The Harrisburg campus focuses on cardiology, women and children, and transplant services. The third campus provides general acute care services with particular strengths in orthopedics, neurosciences, rehabilitation, and bariatric surgery.[2]

When Longenderfer assumed the CEO role in 2000, he established *quality and safety* as the number one priority for the system. Clinical consolidation was one initiative toward this end, combining programs with their related volumes, reducing cost, and enhancing clinical skills to improve patient care. Management compensation is tied more to quality and safety outcomes than to financial metrics.[3] The focus on quality has led to Pinnacle being recognized for its cardiovascular, neurology, neurosurgery, and orthopedic services. A recent five-year initiative to reduce surgical infections yielded a 30 percent decrease in cardiac surgical site infections and a 50 percent decrease in orthopedic surgical site infections.[4] These and other results are possible because decisions were made related to the merger that poised the organization for success. Rather than allow the merger to get bogged down in internal politics, past promises, and other legacy issues, leadership established an external focus: to serve the community's patient care needs.

In another case, as mentioned in previous chapters, Health First in Brevard County, located on Florida's "space coast," was formed more than fifteen years ago from the merger of Holmes Regional Medical Center and Cape Canaveral Hospital. The system has grown from $200 million at its inception to more than $1 billion in revenues. It includes three hospitals (with a fourth due to open in 2011), a medical group of more than a hundred physicians, and its own health plan. The health plan serves more than 63,000 residents, and its revenue now exceeds $400 million. When the health industry fad of starting or joining provider-based health plans wore off after the merger mania period of the 1990s, Health First did not exit the insurance business. It believed its own health plan was best for the county it served. The two keys to its success have been (1) capitation, as opposed to fee-for-service revenues to providers, and (2) the size of its physician panel being correlated to the number of members in the health plan.[5] In one magazine survey, the Health First Health Plan was ranked in the top 25 of U.S. health plans.[6]

One example of the benefits its members enjoy is demonstrated by the action the health plan team took in 2004 when Florida was hit by four hurricanes. Plan employees called its members to ensure they were safe and had all their required medications. In the post-hurricane recovery, the cost for Health First Health Plan was lower than that of its competitors.[7] The health plan had the flexibility to act fast in the interest of its members and community.

As previously discussed, and as summarized in figure 6-1, mergers can fail for any number of reasons.

In the remainder of this chapter we examine the common characteristics demonstrated by successful mergers.

If success in health care is defined as bringing value to the overall community and to the patients who use hospital services, then what ingredients make a successful merger? The critical success factors in forming mergers are the following:

- Sound business rational
- Mission, vision, and values clearly articulated and embraced
- Commitment to succeed that exceeds the legal form of the merger
- Leadership of management, board, and physicians that brings required skills to succeed
- Strategic business plan that maps out implementation of merger objectives

Compelling Reasons to Merge Translate to Sound Business Rationale

In the for-profit segment of the health care industry, return on shareholder equity is a primary driver of merger and acquisition

Figure 6-1. How to Ensure a Failed Merger

- Compelling reasons to merge do not translate to sound business reasons.
- The CEO is not sure the merger is good for his or her career.
- The management team does not want the merger.
- The board takes management's word that the merger is feasible without asking pertinent questions.
- Board or sponsor commitment is superficial.
- The merger is only about saving money.
- A strategic business plan is produced after the merger.
- "Out" clauses are placed in the agreement in case one party does not like how the merger is progressing.
- The merger is a defensive strategy, with no adequate offensive (strategic) plan.
- The merger is built on relationships, not sound business reasons.
- The assumption is made that culture differences will be easily resolved.
- Two or more weak organizations merge thinking they will become strong together.
- Money will come from the parent or another party and the weak entity will keep its autonomy.
- Co-C-suite roles are established.
- The belief that "50-50" is hardened principle rather than spirit of a transaction.
- The merger is a reaction rather than a sound strategy.
- The medical staffs are merged with no compelling reason to do so.
- The fund-raising arms of the entities are merged too quickly, risking alienation of lifelong contributors.
- Money is saved by skimping on legal and business advice.
- Consultants are hired who tell the organizations only what they want to hear.
- Inexperienced consultants and lawyers are hired.
- The merger is conducted based on the thinking that no antitrust issues will arise in the market.
- The board approves reserve powers without understanding their implications.

activity. Wall Street rewards growth, and organic growth is supplemented or propelled by mergers and acquisitions. The focus is often short term, with quarterly earnings serving as the report card on performance and the business rationale for the merger.

In the not-for-profit segment of the industry, transactions must be based on long-term considerations. A sound business reason has to exist that transcends today's compelling reason (or fad) to merge community-based assets.

In an earlier chapter, we saw how mergers or acquisitions take place because the financial situation of an organization left little choice. Or they occur because the original mission is ended or fulfilled, and the best course for the community is to close the hospital. The for-profit sector has exercised this option well for years, removing excess capacity that other organizations could not bring themselves to do.

In other cases, stand-alone hospitals or small health systems consider mergers because they hope to find a friendly bank in the form of a larger health system and seek to preserve autonomy while taking the cash. Good luck.

As discussed in previous chapters, a number of mergers that were put together in the 1990s as a reaction to fears of managed care capitation, for-profit competitors, or "Hillary Care" fell apart once these fears faded and the merger fad lost its luster. The return to autonomy or the status quo looked like a safe haven.

Executives and trustees must realize that the compelling issues that face hospitals and health systems today may dissipate in a few years. Mergers based on sound business and mission reasons will be better positioned to survive and thrive. The challenge for management and boards is to take a long-term view of the business impact of a potential merger transaction and make prudent decisions on the merits to the organization and the communities served by the proposed merger entities. Sound business reasons are supported by each party's clear objectives and goals for the transaction.

As mentioned in chapter 3, understanding what an organization must achieve from a transaction is imperative to its long-term success. Merger objectives and principles are important underpinnings of future success; they help guide the organization to evaluate merger or acquisition opportunities and, importantly, to be able to walk away from a transaction that does not live up to its merger objectives and principles.

One of the founding executives of Catholic Health Initiatives (CHI) reflects in hindsight that the compelling reason for entering into the transaction with two other systems—for-profit encroachment on Catholic health care—was likely exaggerated; however, he also views the combined merged organization as greater today than the pre-merger organizations could have ever been if they had continued as separate entities.[8] The transaction was undergirded by sound business and mission rationale.

Recall that at the time the CHI merger was being contemplated, several for-profit systems had evolved into national companies. The formation of some larger for-profit systems in the 1980s to mid-1990s gave the industry its first view of delivery systems on a national level. The formation of CHI in 1996 was the first significant not-for-profit response to the for-profit national health care systems. As this founding CEO put it, "It was not only a leap frog strategy, it was a giant leap." A long-term view was taken from the initial planning of the three-system merger, with goals set for the first five and ten years post-merger.[9] The long-term mission and business focus of the transaction transcended the compelling reasons of the era; thus, the CHI system continues and is now nearing fifteen years of providing Catholic health care services throughout the United States.

Mission, Vision, and Values

Mergers need to be concerned with more than money to succeed. Designation as for-profit or not-for-profit does not matter, and executives and employees need a purpose that goes beyond finances. A merger that is primarily contemplated to save money will excite few people—it is like asking doctors to get excited about helping a hospital cut costs; they may go through the motions, but sustainable results will not prevail. When Ford Motor Company decided to build the Edsel automobile, the Edsel was the best-researched and -engineered car of its era. The only problem was that the people in the company did not believe in it.[10] Consequently, the Edsel endures as a symbol of corporate failure.

Winning the hearts and minds of people takes an overarching purpose that people can embrace. Faith-based organizations perhaps have an advantage, a history of purpose that continues through to the present day. Other secular not-for-profits have engendered commitment by promoting the continued preservation of community-based (not-for-profit) hospital care. For-profit hospitals have sought to demonstrate that the value of process improvement and standardization enhances quality of care while lowering costs to those who pay for the care. Furthermore, paying taxes positions them as valuable community contributors. The bottom line is, the mission, vision, and values need to be clear so that people look outward at the opportunities, not inward, worried about what will happen next. An outward focus that generates the behavior change needed to accomplish the mission is the essence of culture building. Peter Drucker notes that effective mission and vision statements need three components:[11]

- *Competence*: Look at the strength of the merged organization and build on this strength.
- *Opportunities*: Given the limited resources of people and money, and based on organizational competence, where are the opportunities to make a difference and set a new standard? Just as important, identify those areas that the organization should no longer be involved in and shift resources to other opportunities. Not-for-profit organizations in particular find it difficult to let go, thus compromising resources needed for new opportunities.

- *Commitment*: Organizational and personal/professional commitment underlie strategic and operational success. Any number of mergers or strategies (for instance, building a provider-owned health plan) failed for lack of true belief or commitment.

Where there is commitment, there is organizational power to succeed in the marketplace. After the formation of Catholic Health Initiatives, patience with and understanding of the feelings of stakeholders' at each facility were in evidence when the mission statement of both CHI and the individual facility were displayed for about three years while the reality and vision of the new sponsor took hold.[12] Commitment calls for time and patience in building a culture.

At Health First, so many of the employees have more than twenty years of service that no hall in Brevard County is big enough to hold them all.[13] At Texas Health Resources, the 19,000 employees share in the performance success of the organization in the form of bonuses. Now seeking to achieve the Malcolm Baldrige National Quality Award in the Health Care Category, the organization's employees, management, and board have a stake in improved outcomes and better service.[14] Systems that can provide a vision that is understood and embraced, combined with a career track and reward system for outstanding service and performance, gain a human capital advantage.

It's the Commitment, Not the Legal Model

The form of legal model has little to do with the success or failure of hospital mergers. Some observers contend that legal models that are less than full-asset mergers are setting themselves up for future failure. For example, in January 2009, Christ Hospital reached agreement with the Health Alliance in Cincinnati, Ohio, for terms of its departure from the system, thus avoiding a legal confrontation in the court system.[15] The Health Alliance is not a full-asset merger.

Successful mergers have been formed by joint operating agreements (JOAs), such as BayCare Health System and or CHI, the latter of which inherited four JOAs at its beginning.[16]

The legal model of some mergers, such as some in which Bon Secours Health System participated, is the joint venture.[17] Similarly, the initial Morton Plant Mease merger, discussed in earlier chapters, was a joint venture for its first ten years in response to an antitrust consent order. Interestingly, this organization has had merger experience under three different legal models—the joint venture, a full merger as Morton Plant Mease, and a joint operating agreement as part of the BayCare Health System— and has been successful under all three.

On the other hand, mergers thought to have been ironclad have failed and broken up. One executive described a merger in which his entity owned 90 percent of the merged organization with performance milestones that would eventually lead that organization to own all of it; however, the perceived culture differences and disagreements over financial commitments within the first year of the merger led to its eventual demise. *A full-asset merger will certainly be more difficult to break up, but on the other hand, a full-asset merger does not guarantee success.*

The 1992 presidential campaign between George H.W. Bush and Bill Clinton came to be characterized by the statement made by Clinton, "It's the economy, stupid." Similarly, although not nearly so straightforward, in mergers, it's not the legal model, it's the commitment.

When Holmes Regional Medical Center was negotiating with Cape Canaveral Hospital, Mike Means remembers, "We burned the life boats." Larry Garrison, then CEO of the smaller Cape Canaveral Hospital, confirms that there would be no looking back, only a commitment to look ahead and make the merger work.[18] No out clauses were incorporated into the merger agreement.

Another chief executive currently in merger negotiations comments that he is not contemplating any out clauses in the proposed merger. He sees his job and that of his team as doing their homework up front.

Thus, one factor that certainly will increase the chances of failure of a merger is the placement of out clauses in the agreement. Out clauses are upfront expressions of the lack of commitment before the merger even commences. Eventually one party will find a reason to get out. In the University of California, San Francisco Medical Center (UCSF) and Stanford University Health merger, the agreement permitted either UCSF or Stanford to petition for an involuntary dissolution from the not-for-profit public benefit corporation that formed the legal model of the merger.[19] The failed merger of St. Vincent and Baptist hospitals, located in Jacksonville, Florida, was facilitated by an out clause.[20] We saw in an earlier chapter that the de-merger in Huntington, West Virginia, between Cabell and St. Mary's hospitals was helped by a clause in the agreement that a party wishing to leave the arrangement could make a prescribed payment, the amount of which was thought at the time to be sufficiently prohibitive in a practical sense from any party exercising this clause.[21]

Finally, Robert Issai, president and CEO of the Daughters of Charity Health System, comments that the publicity of the breakup in 2001 of his system from Catholic Healthcare West after six years generated a number of calls inquiring about how to get out of mergers, which in itself is telling. His counsel to such callers is, "Does your organization have $25 million of cash lying around it doesn't know what to do with?"[22] Breaking up mergers is exponentially more expensive than putting them together. Assuring the commitment, business rationale, adherence to ground rules, and understanding of the workings of the transaction is considered essential upfront work. If it is gray, walk away.

On the other hand, mergers have survived and in fact thrived despite any number of legal and marketplace challenges. Understanding and commitment, not the legal model, will undergird the success of the transaction.

Leadership

One hallmark of mergers that succeed is the selection of appropriate and well-suited leaders of the new entity. Factors that characterize successful mergers in the area of leadership include appropriate CEO and board selection, management stability, and a culture of accountability.

Chief Executive Officer and Board Selection

There is no such thing as a 50-50 merger. Someone has to be in charge, or the merged organization will fail. In some cases, keeping the merging CEOs together, but in different positions in a merged organization, has worked well; in other cases, keeping multiple former executives in different roles has not worked and in fact has impeded the progress of the merger.[23,24]

Regardless of which organization assumes the lead, the selection of the CEO is critical. He or she becomes the culture cornerstone of the new organization (see chapter 4) and carries out the policies of the newly merged board.

"The foundation of effective leadership is thinking through the organization's mission, defining and establishing it, clearly and visibly. The leader sets the goals, sets the priorities, and sets and maintains the standards." Furthermore, "What distinguishes the leader from the misleader are his goals. Whether the compromises he makes with the constraints of reality—which may involve political, economic, financial or people problems— are compatible with his mission and goals or lead away from them determines whether he is an effective leader."[25]

The challenge for the merged board is to make sure it has the right leader. That person may be hired from outside the organization. Whether to go outside or stay inside for the selection of CEO is a difficult call for hospital boards. Most boards in merger discussions have their own favorite internal candidate. The question is, can the merged entity's chief executive rally people from different organizations, different histories, and different cultures to focus on a greater good that engenders the trust and responses required to achieve the goals of the merged organization? For that executive who is, in fact, the internal favored candidate, he or she needs to think long and hard about whether his or her leadership, passion, vision, integrity, and communication skills will transcend whatever today's and yesterday's successes, political connections, or even charisma might bring to the deal.

Management Team Stability

The size and complexity of the merged organization matter. It speaks to the kind of management capability the merged organization will need going forward. Success as a chief financial officer of one or two community hospitals does not automatically translate into having the capability to run a billion dollar health care enterprise. Though a blending of executives from different organizations becomes necessary to create a culture of partnership versus that of a takeover, the challenge for the chief executive and board is to thoughtfully consider the skill sets required to manage the merged enterprise and place personal agendas and political expediency on the back burner.

The skill sets that got us to the present day may have brought us success, but the executive skills needed to move a merged organization even further might require different skills. Determining accurately these required skills will help to identify the type of executives needed to position the merged entity for success. One search consultant makes it a point to ask board members to describe the leadership skills that brought the organization its current success. Then he asks them what skills will be needed for a merged organization; often board members begin to realize that those skill sets might require a different leader.[26]

One indicator of the success of executive selection in mergers is the management stability that remains in place ten and fifteen years post-merger, as demonstrated at organizations such as Sentara, Health First, BayCare, California Pacific Medical Center, and Sutter Health, to name a few. In these organizations the key executives selected to serve in the merged organization at its inception are still in senior positions of leadership a decade and more later, and importantly, each organization is performing well. Performance counts; results matter. Management stability is earned.

Accountability

Effective leaders adhere to standards, and their conduct sets the example for others to follow. Others in the organization, when observing such leaders, use the word *integrity* to describe their character. These leaders hold themselves and others accountable for their performance and for their actions, an integral component of achieving the merger's goals and cultivating a culture in which people embrace the vision and goals.

Given that mergers take years to gain traction, particularly in areas such as clinical consolidation, branding, and culture, organizations should consider developing an annual report on merger progress and efficiencies. Sometimes merger efficiencies are tracked because the merger was subject to legal agreement by state or federal officials to document savings for a certain period of time. However, absent such mandatory requirements, the effectiveness of other mergers is not rigorously tracked. Has the merger achieved what it was designed to achieve in meeting major merger objectives? How specifically have the patients and community benefited? Are the board and management holding themselves accountable for achieving the outcomes they stated would be accomplished? Words might sound good and read well for a short time on the Internet and in hard print, but our actions reveal our priorities, focus, and commitment.

An annual report card for a period of five to ten years (figure 6-2) should provide focus on achieving merger goals. One executive noted that a report card look-back exercise helped his organization move from a frustrating 51 percent–49 percent partnership to a full merger, which, in turn, provided a new hospital for his community.[27]

Not every aspect of a merger will proceed as anticipated in achieving benefits. Furthermore, executives will make their

Figure 6-2. Tracking Merger Outcomes: Annual Report Card

Establish metrics and milestones as part of strategic plan and annual budgets: • Cost savings   • Capital avoidance   • Improved access/service distribution   • Clinical enhancements/consolidation   • Key strategic investments
What are our critical success factors (specific, measurable)?
For each area, what is working, and what is not working?   • Governance   • Management   • Operations   • Clinical/medical staff   • Financials   • Service/culture   • Fund-raising   • Branding

own mistakes. The effective leaders admit to them and correct them in a timely manner. Mistakes will happen; the response to them is what sets an effective management team apart. As Martin Brotman, MD, CEO of California Pacific Medical Center, stated, "If an executive hire is not a fit, admit it and fix it quickly as possible."[28]

Another executive team mentioned its organization's efforts to make a modest reduction of benefits a decade ago when the merged organization encountered a brief financial challenge. What seemed like a reasonable reduction to management was not viewed as such by the employees, causing a significant disruption. In reflecting on what management sought to achieve, they realized their mistake and admitted it, understanding policies are also drivers of culture. The informal leaders within the organization appreciated the candid response and put much effort into getting relationships back on track in the organization. The leader who can appropriately place blame at his or her own feet will be in a better position to hold others accountable for performance.

Strategy as It Affects Patient Care and Outcomes

Bad culture eats strategy. Many executives understand this. But just as importantly, they must understand that bad strategy trumps mergers. A merger has to make business sense, and it has to make clinical sense; that is, it needs to make patient care sense. One goal of the UCSF-Stanford merger in 1997 was to quickly integrate service lines, and this effort became one of a number of contributing factors to its demise after two years. The leadership team felt it had twelve to eighteen months to achieve this integration. Perhaps in hindsight it would have chosen a more deliberate approach, selecting areas of integration where mutual strength and working relationships existed, as in children services, such that success in one area may have provided a better platform for integration in other areas.[29]

In the PinnacleHealth case noted at the beginning of this chapter, the decision to consolidate clinical services was at the outset considered best for patient care, efficiency, and cost. However, the organization moved deliberately, taking obstetric services from one campus and consolidating it on another campus. The CEO of Pinnacle counsels, however, that when consolidating services to another campus, take steps to be sure they cannot be moved back. Reconfigure the old space; do not leave it as it was, because if it is empty, the politicking will only grow to bring that service back.[30]

For patient care, clearly the movement toward sharing best practices produces better outcomes of care and reduces the cost of that care. One chief medical officer noted that his system examined four areas (urinary tract infections, ulcers, falls, and deep vein thrombosis) and learned it had a $150 million opportunity to reduce variation of care. Achieving even 50 percent of this expectation would significantly benefit patient outcomes and cost.[31]

Merger efficiencies and the primary benefits to be derived are components of a strategic plan that translates to better patient care and outcomes (table 6-1).

In mergers that took significant time and cost to gain traction, a business or strategic plan developed *before* the merger took place should have provided sufficient information to indicate the chances of success of the merger as well as the impediments (such as service consolidation) it would likely encounter. The lack of a strategic business plan before close, or the inability to even consider it because it might kill the deal, are red flags waiting for someone to call attention to the rationale for the merger in the first place.

An organization that had merged in the late 1990s attempted a leap frog strategy with a competitor in developing cardiology services, including initiating open heart services, to compete with a larger hospital. Though the merger made sense, the cardiology strategy implemented was seen by medical staff leaders as lacking in depth and breadth of services. To their view, the required investment of funds was not made, including failing to recruit the best physicians to compete with the larger hospital. Ultimately, the strategy failed, as physicians continued to refer patients to the competing hospital that enjoyed a very good reputation for such services. The resulting financial fallout from the failed strategy proved to be terminal. The hospital could not recover from it, and its faith-based parent sold it to a for-profit hospital company. In short, bad strategy ate the merger.

This case brings up an important point in considering strategic initiatives. Executives, especially financial executives, are accustomed to thinking about "opportunity cost," weighing the benefits of a strategic initiative versus other opportunities that might be forgone. However, executives need to be more

Table 6-1. Targeted Patient/Community Benefits of Mergers

Merger Efficiency	Primary Benefit
Less executive/middle management	Cost
Back-office consolidation	Cost
Capital avoidance (duplicative)	Cost
Purchasing/supply chain efficiencies	Cost/quality
Improved access to capital	Cost
Improved cash management/treasury functions	Cost/income
Improved geographic distribution: • Ambulatory/clinics • Urgent care • Freestanding emergency rooms • Physician recruitment/placement • Specialty hospitals	Access
Education: • Patient information classes: on-site and Web based • Health screenings • Medical education: more robust	Access/quality
Technology investment focused/prioritized: • Electronic health record • Expensive, high-tech equipment	Cost/quality
Reduce variation in patient outcomes: • Sharing of better/best practices • Improve safety • Reduce readmissions/infections	Quality/cost

Clinical consolidation:
• Improve volumes at specific locations
• Improve volumes for critical services, e.g.:
  —Pediatrics
  —Neonatal intensive care unit
  —Trauma
  —Air ambulance
• Improve clinical skills
• Further ability to improve outcomes/service
	Quality/cost

sensitive when weighing opportunities versus risk. Risk needs to be thought of as the *cost of failure*. If a contemplated objective (for instance, entering into a merger agreement, integrating a service line, launching a new program, or embarking on a comprehensive information system upgrade) fails, what happens? Can the organization absorb the consequences of the failure, or will it lead to the organization's demise? Is an exit strategy in place? A merger and acquisition executive with experience in for-profit and not-for profit companies noted in his experience that the for-profit hospitals always have an exit strategy, while the not-for-profits tend not to have one.[32]

If a strategic mistake can be absorbed by the organization (meaning it does not take the organization down), the question then becomes, What other organizational projects and initiatives currently in play or under consideration will need to be delayed or halted to recover from a failed strategy? Thinking about opportunities and weighing them against the risk and cost of partial or total failure will help the management team make prudent strategic decisions.

Physicians at the Planning Table

Physicians may not have the same influence to back or block hospital mergers as they did a decade or more ago. This loss of influence is due in part to the fact that physicians have taken revenue from hospitals, so they are competitors in a number of venues. Furthermore, physicians have formed into groups and super groups for revenue and cost-containment reasons. As a result, their activities will increasingly be on the radar screen of antitrust regulators, thus physicians are gaining some appreciation as to why hospitals merge. Yet other physicians are increasingly becoming hospital employees.

The challenge for hospital executives is to decide whether physicians are their competitor, client, customer, or partner, or perhaps a combination of all these. Ultimately, however, when it comes to patient outcomes and community benefit, physicians need to be partners with the merged entity. One chief medical officer disputes the notion that all health care is local, noting it flies in the face of data. Tools provided with electronic medical records, such as built-in order sets, provide clinical prompts for the physicians and better monitoring of care processes.[33] To create a culture of improved patient outcomes, including clinical consolidation, physicians must have significant and ongoing involvement in strategic planning for successful organizational and patient care outcomes.

Financial Planning—and Action

A strong balance sheet and strong market share allow an organization to be poised for opportunity. Stating the obvious, cash flow fuels the organization to carry out its mission of patient care. Profits are required if the organization is to be viable and competitive—and in a position to take advantage of opportunities. Operating and capital budgets are the annual implementation tactics of the organization's overall strategic plan. In successful mergers, a high correlation exists between the annual operating/financial plan and the organization's strategic plan. Without this relationship, the strategic plan lacks relevance. Also a factor in successful mergers is a complete understanding of the ground rules of capital allocation. Amazingly, in some hospitals the view still prevails that capital comes from "corporate," not realizing that capital is a function of the sum of the parts; the money comes from the members, not vice versa.

Weak-performing organizations within a system negatively affect cash flow and compromise the capital needs of other entities in the system. Corrective and timely action is necessary; if resolution cannot be obtained, either an exit strategy is required or a mission decision is made to keep the weak-performing asset. Either decision has implications for the allocation of resources and talent within the system, and those implications need to be communicated and understood by stakeholders. Otherwise, weak links in a system will have a demoralizing effect on other system members. Are your best people spending time on problems, or on taking advantage of opportunities? Remember, bad strategy, including weak performers, eats mergers.

Branding as a Component of Strategy

What to name a merged entity is another sensitive issue in mergers. As one former board chair relayed, he never forgot the advice of a consultant who counseled him that three factors usually cause mergers to fail, and none had to do with the business merits: selecting the CEO, forming the new board, and naming the merged entity.[34] With system formation, branding a corporate name has become a challenge and an opportunity. As hospitals and health systems are fairly new to the world of corporate mergers, the experiences of several organizations are worth considering.

When Alta Bates of Sutter in Berkeley, California, merged with Summit Medical Center of Oakland, the CEO was appreciative that Sutter's CEO did not force an immediate name change, understanding that Alta Bates had a legacy of a hundred years in the Berkeley community. The merged entity became known as Alta Bates Summit.[35] Another executive believes corporate branding is meaningless: Why compromise hospital brand names that have been around for decades or perhaps a hundred years or more?[36]

Nevertheless, as the hospital industry continues to consolidate into systems, the use and branding of corporate names will likely increase, but it is not as easy a process as it may seem. When the PROMINA Health System, in Atlanta, was formed, the name was intended to infer prominence.[37] However, one former PROMINA executive commented that the name took on a negative connotation. Chosen with the help of a consultant, the name came to invoke the idea of "preeminence," as in taking over everything.[38] Furthermore, local hospitals were free to decide how to use the corporate name. Some hospitals put the corporate name at the top of their signage and letterhead, while others put it at the bottom. This inconsistency led to debates among the hospital leaders as to which members were more committed to the system.[39]

The formation and name Health First (Holmes Regional and Cape Canaveral in Florida) came about because the CEO of Cape Canaveral bought a group of urgent care centers from the physician owners and bought the name "Health First" along with it—a name registered in Florida. In contemplating the merger, the CEO of Holmes liked it and the decision was made to use it. However, confusion arose with the public, particularly with the name being connected to the Health First Health Plan; the perception was that a commercial company had taken over the hospitals. The public was not the only group confused; physicians were, as well. In response, the hospital names are now displayed prominently, with Health First as a byline. In the years since the 1994 merger, the name has become better known and is now a significant asset, particularly in areas such as private-duty nursing and home health. Patients' familiarity with the name engenders a sense of safety and confidence. The CEO and chief operating officer (COO) note they would not have changed their decision on the corporate name, but they should have spent considerably more time in educating stakeholders.[40]

In the Cabell–St Mary's merger in Huntington, West Virginia, the branding of a system name came from a board member who suggested "Genesis" as the merged hospitals were embarking on a new beginning in 1998. The first attempt was to call it Genesis Healthcare System, but it became confused with a nursing home chain, so the name was later changed to Genesis Hospital System.[41] Another executive believes the corporate branding was one more step toward diffusing the previous decades of competitive culture between the two hospitals; however, he observed that the Catholic sponsor became concerned that the branding was redefining its ministry, given the name St. Mary's is integral to the overall ministry, and it did not want this name to "fade."[42] Regardless of naming attempts to facilitate a new beginning, the merger ended after four years.

As one can see from these examples, branding is a complicated issue. For hospital systems, it is clearly a work in progress.

The CEO of Sutter notes that in terms of branding, the system name is "not over the hill yet." Though in most markets after many years the Sutter name is top of mind, he notes in areas such as San Francisco, its own member hospital, California Pacific Medical Center, still enjoys top-of-mind name awareness.[43]

As one executive put the discussion in perspective, how many people know that Godiva Chocolatier, a strong brand name, is owned by Campbell Soup Company?[44] Hospital names have been embedded in our communities for many years. Corporate branding with new names will take time to be effective.

Texas Health Resources, twelve years into a merger at the time of this writing, just in the past year came out with a corporate logo after comprehensive testing. The CEO notes that credibility and timing are important to branding corporate names and the strategy associated with it.[45]

Steve Mason, current CEO of BayCare Health System, believes the success of future mergers rides on much more than the hospitals themselves. In integrating other components of health care, such as physicians, ambulatory care, and nursing home services, branding will be important in the minds of customers to identify and associate value and expertise in health care. He recently hired a senior executive of marketing from a corporate non–health care company where branding and advertising is aimed at producing a revenue stream and using technology, such as social networks, to understand what patients want and need to win them to his organization.[46]

In summary, although it seems obvious, it bears emphasizing that successful mergers require a lot of effort and teamwork. While getting a deal done requires time, money, focus, and perseverance, the real work begins the day the merger is consummated.

A community and its patients benefit from the dedication and commitment put forth to achieve merger goals. A successful merger will realize economies of scale, thus reducing cost. The more substantive opportunity is to share clinical knowledge and improve processes that lead to better patient care; in addition, where geographically possible, consolidating services will further enhance clinical skill sets, quality, and outcomes of care.

Figure 6-3 lists the actions required by management and the board to enhance the chances of a merger to provide better service and competitive cost for its patients and community.

Figure 6-3. Salient Features of Successful Mergers

Pre-merger Planning
- Compelling reasons to merge
- Sound business reason to merge
- Clearly articulated merger objectives
- Development of criteria to evaluate merger merits
- Opportunity (financials, capital access, patient services) that exceeds risk/cost of failure
- Understanding of advantages: Each party knows and understands what it brings to the table
- Recognizing impediments: Each party understands the baggage it brings to the table
- Communication plan development
- Development of strategic business plan prior to close/updated after close: identify essentials
- Thorough execution of due diligence

Post-Closing Execution
- Board commitment to "oneness," best interest of new organization
- Clearly written mission, vision, values: people can understand/ embrace
- Chief executive's capability to carry out mission, vision, values
- Senior management team's possession of skills need to make merger successful
- Physicians' involvement in strategic planning
- Physicians' leadership in clinical consolidation and outcomes improvement
- Effective communication/branding strategy
- Establishment of culture pillars: measurement, monitoring, accountability, communication
- Commitment to make the merger work superseding the legal model
- A merger business model that facilitates better patient care outcomes and service

References

1. Roger Longenderfer, MD, president and CEO, PinnacleHealth System, interview with author, Harrisburg, Pennsylvania, August 3, 2009.
2. Ibid.
3. Ibid.
4. Pinnacle Health, "Hospital Infection Rates" [http://www.pinnacle health.org/?/quality-of-care-infection-rates]. Accessed October 7, 2009.
5. Michael Means, CEO, and Larry Garrison, COO, Health First, interview with author, Rockledge, Florida, June 24, 2009.
6. Health First, "Health First Health Plans Ranked One of Top 25 in the Nation" [http://www.health-first.org/news_and_events/hfhp_us_news_2008.cfm]. Accessed October 2, 2009.
7. Means and Garrison interview.
8. Ronald R. Aldrich, former CEO, Franciscan Health System, interview with author, Hope, Idaho, June 29, 2009.
9. Ibid.
10. Peter F. Drucker, *Managing the Nonprofit Organization* (New York: HarperCollins, 1990), 7.
11. Ibid., 7–8.
12. Patricia A. Cahill and Maryanna Coyle, *Catholic Health Initiatives, a Spirit of Innovation, a Legacy of Care, the Early Years* (Denver: Catholic Health Initiatives, 2006), 144.
13. Means and Garrison interview.
14. Douglas D. Hawthorne, CEO, Texas Health Resources, interview with author, Arlington, Texas, September 21, 2009.
15. *Modern Healthcare* Alerts, "Christ Hospital Reaches Agreement to Avoid Legal Battle" [http://www.alerts@ModernHealthcare.com]. Accessed January 12, 2009.
16. Hawthorne interview.
17. John Shea, senior vice president, Development, and senior vice president, Sponsorship, Bon Secours Health System, interview with author, Marriottsville, Maryland, July 7, 2009.
18. Means and Garrison interview.
19. John A. Kastor, *Mergers of Teaching Hospitals in Boston, New York, and Northern California* (Ann Arbor, MI: University of Michigan Press, 2003), 281.
20. Anthony J. Filer, senior system vice president and chief financial officer, Provena Health System, interview with author, Mokena, Illinois, August 20, 2009.
21. J. Thomas Jones, president and CEO, West Virginia United Health System, interview with author, Fairmont, West Virginia, July 10, 2009.

22. Robert Issai, president and CEO, Daughters of Charity Health System, interview with author, Los Altos Hills, California, July 21, 2009.
23. Filer interview.
24. William T. Foley, CEO, Cook County Health System and Hospitals, interview with author, Chicago, August 19, 2009.
25. Peter F. Drucker, *Managing for the Future: The 1990's and Beyond* (New York: Dutton, 1992), 121.
26. John Ferry, MD, senior client partner, Korn Ferry International, interview with author, Boston, November 11, 2009.
27. Les A. Donahue, CEO, St. Thomas Hospital and former CEO, Virginia Beach and Williamsburg hospitals as part of Sentara, interview with author, Nashville, Tennessee, October 9, 2009.
28. Martin Brotman, MD, CEO, California Pacific Medical Center, interview with author, San Francisco, July 22, 2009.
29. William J. (Bill) Kerr, former CEO, University of California, San Francisco Medical Center, and former COO, UCSF Stanford Health Care, interview with author, San Francisco, September 22, 2009.
30. Longenderfer interview.
31. Terrence O'Rourke, MD, chief medical officer, Trinity Health, and former board chair and CMO, Centura Health, interview with author, Novi, Michigan, August 12, 2009.
32. Shea interview.
33. O'Rourke interview.
34. Alan Bomstein, former board chair, Morton Plant and Morton Plant Mease, interview with author, Clearwater, Florida, November 2, 2009.
35. Warren Kirk, CEO, Alta Bates Summit Medical Center, interview with author, Oakland, California, July 22, 2009.
36. Thomas Beeman, PhD, CEO, Lancaster General Health, interview with author, Lancaster, Pennsylvania, July 13, 2009.
37. Bernard L. (Bernie) Brown, CEO (retired), PROMINA Health, interview with author, Atlanta, July 16, 2009.
38. Bonnie Phipps, CEO, St. Agnes Hospital, and former CEO, PROMINA Health, interview with author, Baltimore, Maryland, July 1, 2009.
39. Brown interview.
40. Means and Garrison interview.
41. Jones interview.
42. Michael Sellards, CEO, St. Mary's Hospital and Palatine Health System, interview with author, Huntington, West Virginia, July 9, 2009.

43. Patrick Fry, CEO, Sutter Health, interview with author, Sacramento, California, July 20, 2009.
44. Longenderfer interview.
45. Hawthorne interview.
46. Steven R. Mason, CEO, BayCare Health System, and former COO, Texas Health Resources, interview with author, Clearwater, Florida, September 28, 2009.

7

The Future:
From the Benefit of Hindsight

The previous chapters review cases of hospital mergers that have been successful not only in financial terms but also in terms of improving patient care by sharing data and knowledge and consolidating clinical services to enhance professional skills.

The chapters also present cases in which mergers failed for a variety of reasons: The compelling reasons for merging turned out to be based on a reaction to perceived market conditions rather than on a proactive, sound business case; culture differences were grossly underestimated; or dysfunctional leadership (board or management) looked more inward to protect legacies than outward to envision a better model for patient care access, cost, and outcomes.

The number of mergers over the last ten years, though not insignificant, has slowed from its frenzied pace of the mid-1990s, which averaged approximately 150 per year between 1994 and 1998. The ensuing ten years, from 1999 to 2008, saw an average of sixty mergers a year. For the most recent year, 2009, the number of deals closed during the year was fifty-two, somewhat fewer than the annual average for the previous ten years.[1] Once the compelling drivers of mergers in the mid-1990s dissipated, the hospital industry enjoyed a decade of relative stability and profitability.

As recent as 2007, hospitals experienced record profits, amounting to $43 billion and creating the largest single-year jump in profit margins in at least fifteen years.[2]

The Health Care Environment Has Changed Again

But how the world has changed once again. Less than a year after announcing record profits, hospitals' median profit margins had fallen to zero, with half the hospitals losing money, and median days cash on hand had fallen to historic lows.[3]

The global financial crisis that began in 2008 caused investment portfolios to suffer significant losses, compromising investment and expansion plans of hospitals and health systems, as operating cash became tight and access to credit markets became even tighter. In the third quarter of 2009, total loan balances by lenders fell by the largest margins since data collection began twenty-five years ago, indicating that banks remain reluctant to lend, despite the hundreds of billions of dollars of government bailout money spent to prop up ailing banks.[4] The effect of the recession on individuals has also affected hospitals and physicians, as more than half of Americans indicated they cut back on health care due to cost concerns,[5] with unemployment near 10 percent nationally further driving individual health care decisions. Furthermore, for many employers and employees, health insurance has become too expensive to carry,[6] which negatively affects hospitals, physicians, and insurers. Small businesses in particular have been affected. Those businesses with fewer than 500 employees generated 60 to 80 percent of the net new jobs annually in the United States over the last decade, employing half of all private-sector employees and hiring approximately 40 percent of high-technology workers,[7] such as scientists, engineers, and computer programmers. The recent recession was caused in part by the creation of too few new private-sector jobs in the last decade (table 7-1).

The growth in government jobs in the last decade (where such jobs tend to be consumers of wealth, not creators of

Table 7-1.   U.S. Employment Growth (in millions), 1981–2009

	Government	Private	Total
Reagan years (1981–89)	2,266	14,487	16,753
Bush Sr. years (1989–93)	1,153	1,214	2,367
Clinton years (1993–2001)	–1,795	20,498	18,703
Bush Jr. years (2001–09)	4,146	175	4,321

Source: Bureau of Labor Statistics (not seasonally adjusted); Green Drake Partners LLC.

wealth) and current concerns that U.S. recovery from the recent recession will lack private-sector job growth will carry implications for health care and the overall economy well into the next decade. One reputable reporter and author has characterized the current period as "welcome to the lean years." He goes on to say that the job of leadership now is to close or to downsize services, programs, and personnel, further commenting, "we've gone from the age of government handouts to the age of citizen givebacks, from the age of companions fly free to the age of paying for each bag."[8]

Cost and Quality Continue to Be Issues

Concerns over the cost and quality of health care continue to make headlines across the Internet and in traditional newspapers. Health care spending at the beginning of the 2000 decade stood at $1.4 trillion and, by 2009, had risen to $2.5 trillion. The cost of a family health insurance plan in 2008 is $12,680, double the cost at the beginning of the decade.[9,10] Certainly an aging population is an underlying cause of this growth, but one of the prominent drivers of rising medical cost is the increasing use of new technology.[11] How many magnetic resonance imaging machines are located in any given town, city, or county? The United States leads the world in this count, having the highest number of units per million population among the twenty-nine industrialized nations that comprise the Organisation for Economic Co-operation and Development.

How many computerized tomography scanners are in operation in your market area? The United States has 34.3 million scanners per million compared with an average of 20.2 per million for other industrialized nations.

The total spending on health care as a percentage of gross domestic product is highest in the United States, exceeding 17 percent, nearly double the average of other industrialized countries.[12,13] And in the very near future, by 2012, more than half of U.S. health care spending will be publicly financed, as the trailing effects of the recession on individuals and businesses leave more patients with safety net insurance.[14]

Furthermore, hardly a day goes by without headlines in newspapers or on Web sites featuring stories calling into question the quality of treatment of care. The front page of a national newspaper runs a headline about the "double failure at USA hospitals," speaking of readmission rates and the death rates in hospitals from heart failure and pneumonia.[15] Another large metropolitan newspaper runs a lead headline questioning the competency of clinicians associated with a leading academic medical center performing prostate brachytherapy following adverse outcomes.[16] Yet another newspaper runs a story regarding research that questions the benefit of vertebroplasty, a popular spinal surgery procedure.[17] Pennsylvania's Health Care Cost Containment Council has been collecting data longer than any other state. In summer 2009, it released data on open-heart surgery. The headline comparing experiences in Philadelphia note that five area hospitals had surprisingly high open-heart surgery–related death rates. Furthermore, the article notes that in one suburban county, four hospitals had open-heart surgery programs, with each hospital performing fewer than 100 bypasses a year (as of 2007, the last year for which data were available).[18]

The pressure for transparency on quality and outcomes is not going away; it is only picking up more steam, especially given the concerns of cost of care for individuals, families, companies, and the U.S. economy.

Health Care Reform

These concerns over cost of care, access, service levels, and outcomes associated with this outlay of money has triggered a repeat of the 1990s ("Hillary Care") with President Barack Obama's commitment to reform health care. Few would debate the need for some kind of health care reform. How much reform is needed has been the question at the heart of the political debate, but what family does not have heart-wrenching stories of frustration with obtaining or keeping insurance coverage, protracted wait times for doctors' appointments, and less-than-efficient service at hospitals?

The impact of the cost of health care on the economy and the individual consumer can be seen in table 7-2.

While some observers consider that the U.S. economy's troubles are in part due to too much consumer spending, table 7-2 indicates that when removing health care expenditures from the equation, consumer spending has been consistent. The impact of health care cost on individuals has risen significantly over the last thirty years (table 7-3).

Table 7-2.   Consumer Spending in the United States, 1982–2009

Consumer Personal Consumption Expenditures (PCE) in 2009 as Percentage of Gross Domestic Product	72.0%
Consumer PCE *Excluding* Health Care Spending	
1982	57.5%
1992	56.5%
2002	58.5%
June 2009	58.0%
Source: Green Drake Partners LLC.	

The interesting figure in table 7-3 is that the only period of consumer health care spending stability occurred in the 1990s, when the push for aggressive managed care and the fear of government control (Hillary Care) apparently caused health care companies to hold back on price increases.

Just like the march to transparency in terms of quality of care, reform will move ahead, whether it be incremental (the usual national mode of change in the United States) or more significant. And it will have an impact on hospitals and physicians. Interestingly, the compelling reasons that spurred hospital merger mania in the 1990s look eerily similar for the decade of 2010 (table 7-4).

Perhaps one significant difference between the environmental drivers of the 1990s and those of the upcoming decade is the context of the U.S. position in the international economy. The

Table 7-3.   Health Care Cost as Percentage of Personal Consumption Expenditures, 1980–2008

1980	7.0%
1990	10.0%
2000	10.4%
2008	12.4%

Source: Green Drake Partners LLC.

Table 7-4.   Compelling Environmental Drivers for Merger, 1990s versus 2010s

1990s	2010s
Revenue: managed care capitation	Revenue: growing volume organically and/or through mergers/acquisitions
Competition: for-profit hospital growth	Quality of care: transparency to consumer
Reform: "Hillary Care"	Reform: "Obama Care"

United States is a smaller piece of the global economic pie today than it was a decade or more ago, as China, India, and other emerging markets create more competitive pressure. This shift will only serve to ratchet up the pressure on health care cost and price for services, given the effect they have on our economy and on the competitive international position of the United States.

In fact, the current reform dialogue is already having an impact on health care, including hospitals. In the overall health care industry (not just hospitals), mergers of health care entities comprised 30 percent of all U.S. mergers in 2009, versus the usual rate of 10 percent, the principal driver being the efforts to find new revenues. Some segments of the industry are viewed to be certain beneficiaries of federal reform legislation, such as life science research, research laboratories, and health care information technology.[19]

In regard to the last beneficiary, particularly the movement toward transparency and portability of health information, the American Recovery and Reinvestment Act of 2009 provides reimbursement incentives for hospitals and physicians to be meaningful users of electronic health records (EHRs). Most of these reimbursement payments to providers take place between 2011 and 2015.[20] Providers are pushing themselves to be in position to receive these funds by accelerating their clinical transformation efforts. Some do so within the context of sound planning, and others do not. One forward-looking organization, Sentara Healthcare, tracks both the value and return on investment for information technology. It has redesigned eighteen processes of care over the last few years, covering the entire care continuum. In addition, it measures specific improvements in various areas relating to quality, safety, and compliance initiatives and expects a positive internal rate of return on its investment. The organization links technology investment back to its strategic and business objectives.[21]

Others view information technology as infrastructure sunk cost. One consultant lamented over several smaller or mid-sized hospitals he believes unnecessarily signed high-price vendor contracts, rather than pursuing more economical choices, convinced the availability of federal stimulus money facilitated unwise business decisions that may eventually cost chief information officers and perhaps other senior managers their jobs.[22] The government incentives are aimed at jump-starting a health care industry that lags far behind the technology capabilities of banks, airlines, and retail businesses.

A survey taken in 2008 and published in 2009 indicates that only 9 percent of hospitals have electronic health records.[23] Proponents believe the benefits of EHR systems will improve patient safety and care; however, cost is a major concern. One reason for the stimulus package, then, is the industry's lack of an established return on investment or value of investment on electronic technology.

Efforts to "reform" health care will also need to consider the impact on physicians, which in turn will affect hospitals—and consumers. With some projecting a shortage of 44,000 adult general care physicians, and an overall shortage of 125,000 physicians, by 2025,[24] the implications of expanded coverage under reform become more daunting. By 2025, the number of people over age sixty-five will increase from its current level of 39 million to 64 million. Furthermore, by the end of the next decade (2020), one-third of the physicians currently practicing are expected to have retired.[25] A shortage of physician specialists will also have an impact, as, for example, an insufficient number of pediatricians trained in neurology, gastroenterology, and developmental behaviors has the potential to affect access to care for severely ill children.[26]

Primary care physicians have been feeling the income squeeze for some time now and are seeking alternative measures to increase their income or decrease practice costs. Some are trying the concierge service model, with patients paying significant up-front fees in exchange for flexible access and more time with their physician. However, even this model is not always financially secure. Another approach taken by primary care physicians feeling the economic pinch is to send an annual letter to patients asking them for a voluntary surcharge payment to defray practice expenses and keep the practice viable (see Appendix C). The more likely trend is that physicians will seek the security of a paycheck and become hospital and health system employees. Others will look to merge smaller practices into larger group settings. Hospitals will need to define their relationship with various forms of physician practice models in order to grow revenue.

Challenges related to nurse staffing will continue, with some observers expecting the shortage to exceed 20 percent in the next decade.[27] The ability to recruit and retain physicians and nurses in the upcoming decade will separate growing hospitals and systems from those that are mediocre or going out of business.

The rest of the labor force will also provide management challenges in an era of reform. A recent report from the American Hospital Association suggests that the growing labor shortage is such that health care executives need to accept this reality and start adapting now.[28] With the Democratic Party, currently in power, being an important supporter of unions and with health care considered to be one of the few growth industries, executives can expect to deal with more union challenges. Currently in the United States, only about 11 percent of health care workers are unionized. In Canada, where health care is mostly government controlled, 61 percent of health care workers belong to a union.[29] If this is the direction hospital labor forces take, perhaps hospitals or health systems that have merged and are struggling with clinical service consolidation due to internal pushback might want to consider some urgency in accelerating those initiatives that are better for patient care. The climate won't get easier, so do it now.

Implications for Hospitals and Health Systems

Can your hospital or health system double its revenue in the next decade? Think about the cost of labor (recruitment,

retention, turnover, and benefits), electronic clinical transformation, physician employment and partnerships, supplies,
energy, the greening of hospitals, insurance, debt obligations,
and capital commitments. The need for more revenues to offset
the cost of reform ($155 billion over the next decade pledged
in hospital savings), quality, compliance, growth plans, and
everyday business will provide significant challenges for executives and boards in the next decade. Now add to this the cash
needed to manage surprises. For instance, what if the expanded
insurance coverage under reform does not sufficiently cover the
cost of reform the industry has committed to?

The unexpected will come. Take the use of oil and gas
products as another possible operational and financial challenge. Some experts believe we are close to "peak oil," the
concept that the world is reaching its maximum capacity to
produce oil and will soon be faced with gradually diminishing
supplies. Major oil companies are projecting peak dates after
2015. The experts are debating *when* this will happen, not *if* it
will occur.[30] The implications of a decreased oil supply on the
U.S. economy, our hospitals, and our individual lives will be
significant.

For those who think hospitals and health systems are too
big to fail and the government will come to their aid in adverse
circumstances, consider two events with significant health care
implications.

First, recall the impact of Hurricane Katrina, which devas-
tated the U.S. Gulf Coast in 2005. The government's ability to
respond on any level was found wanting, and the implications
for some of the affected hospitals long lasting. Twelve fewer
hospitals are in operation in the New Orleans area as of June
2009, four years following the hurricane.[31]

Second, in 2009, the ability to ship the H1N1 flu vaccine on
a timely basis challenged physician's offices and hospital emergency rooms across the United States. The federal government
invested $2 billion to develop newer, faster methods of vaccine
production but was not ready to respond to a pandemic.[32]

With epidemiology challenged by new germs and infections, emergency room utilization increasing by those who cannot afford preventive care or insurance absent significant health care reform, and security threats to U.S. infrastructure, hospitals and health systems will need to find ways to be profitable *and* have sufficient cash to deal with both opportunities and adverse circumstances. The government will be limited in its ability to respond to major crises, so the health care industry will have to prepare itself rather than rely on support.

Now ask yourself again, what is your organization's ability to increase revenue over the next ten years to cover the cost of doing business and have enough cash to consider opportunities and weather adverse circumstances? Maybe it does not have to double revenues, but what *is* the volume of business required for your organization to remain meaningful and competitive? Can your organization achieve growth requirements organically? If not, is merger a strategic option to be seriously considered?

With these challenges facing the hospital industry, merger activity will increase. It is likely more regional consolidation will take place. Some large national systems will also consolidate. On the not-for-profit side, this trend would contrast with activity during the last ten years, in which no significant system-to-system consolidation took place. Those systems that terminated talks in the recent past because of issues over governance, sponsorship, or choice of CEO will need to reconsider merger as a strategic option to remain competitive and viable. Local systems will seek in-state partnerships and mergers in efforts to seek more economies of scale and revenue sources.

Given that many hospitals are already part of a system, the *number* of mergers may or may not match those of the 1990s, but the number of acquisitions and divestures will likely increase. As one executive notes, mergers are hard to bring together and hard to manage. "Acquisitions are better than mergers. Divestitures are better than bad mergers!"[33] Large systems that have hospitals in locations with little market concentration (and likely financial challenges) and formidable competitors will need to divest some of these hospitals, as capital and operating cash needed to feed viable business units will demand such moves. Swapping of hospitals with other systems (both for-profit and not-for-profit) will continue as organizations seek to have enough local market presence to make a difference clinically and financially.

Figure 7-1 forecasts the merger and acquisition activity for the next five years (2009 to 2014) in the context of historical hospital merger activity previously discussed.

For-profit systems likely will become more active if reform brings expanded insurance coverage. Expect privately held hospital companies, such as Hospital Corporation of America and Vanguard, to go public again.

In some mid-sized towns and counties that currently have, for example, three hospitals, consolidation may occur to two or perhaps only one hospital. For smaller health systems and for those still freestanding, the time to think about a merger is when they have leverage and strength. Holding on and waiting is not a strategy—weakness translates into an acquisition, not a merger.

Hospital closures will likely increase, at least while excess bed capacity remains. Some hospitals and health systems will

Figure 7-1. Hospital Merger and Acquisition Trend (1990–2008) and Forecast (2009–14)

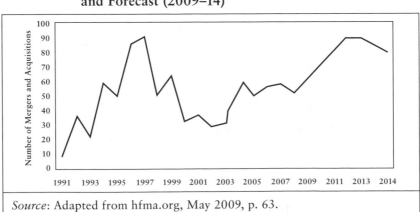

Source: Adapted from hfma.org, May 2009, p. 63.

wait too long to make a merger decision; some have been hanging on far too long already and likely will not survive. One recent survey indicated some executives predict the number of hospitals will decline by 20 percent or more in the next decade.[34] Figure 7-2 summarizes the probable merger activity anticipated in the 2010s.

Size will also be a factor in merger considerations. As one executive put it, bigger is not better, "better is better."[35] The larger systems are challenged to both increase market share and stay connected to executives and staff who face the daily pressures of running a hospital. Corporate executives feel they must drive the changes and standardization required for systems to meet market expectations and mission requirements. Local executives at times feel they are being directed by "corporate" types who have never run a hospital. The dynamic tension is always present but must be balanced so that creativity,

Figure 7-2.   Likely Merger Activity in the Decade of 2010

Mergers	• More local and regional mergers and joint ventures • Increase in system-to-system mergers (national systems)
Divestitures	• Need for more market concentration to justify investment • Financial challenges and distress, money best used elsewhere
Acquisitions	• Someone's divestiture being someone else's opportunity • Freestanding hospitals needing capital and talent • Small systems waiting too long to negotiate a true merger
Closures	• Financial distress too deep to attract buyer • No appreciable market need for services • Politicians no longer able keep it open or find a buyer • Mission over

innovation, and capital allocation foster retention and recruitment of executives who must carry out system objectives and lead organizations through the decade of 2010.

Challenges to the tax-exempt status of not-for-profit health systems could well occur in the next decade. The number of charitable organizations in the United States has increased by 60 percent in just the last decade. Charitable organizations in 2009 cost the government an estimated $50 billion or more in lost tax revenue.[36] Given the sheer size of the federal deficit and the prospect for increased insurance coverage from health reform, hospitals and health systems may provide an easy target for the government to challenge the basis of the tax exemption in an effort to find more tax dollars for a growing government budget.

Thus, governance will need to become more rigorous. Trustees need to better understand underlying enterprise risk and focus on the organization's critical success factors.[37] Does the board know specifically what constitutes its hospital's or system's critical success factors?

No matter if one occupies a corporate position or local provider position, executives and aspiring executives will face significant challenges, which will also present considerable opportunity to demonstrate leadership skills and capabilities.

After all, leadership is about influence. The decade of 2010 will be a time of great challenge and great opportunity for the health care industry. Today, health systems and hospitals need executives who can manage effectively in the context of leading their organizations successfully toward the year 2020.

The mergers, acquisitions, divestitures, and closures in the decade ahead will reposition the health care provider industry. These challenges present opportunities for executives and those who aspire to executive roles specifically in clinical, operational, financial, and administrative areas. The chance to have an impact on the industry is yours to choose. Prepare. Lead. Inspire. Act.

References

1. Vince Galloro and Joe Carlson, "Ready for a Resurgence," *Modern Healthcare* (January 18, 2010): 21–27.
2. *Modern Healthcare*, "U.S. Hospitals Saw Record Profits in '07," *Modern Healthcare* Alert [http://www.alerts@modernHealthcare.com]. Accessed November 7, 2008.
3. HFMA News, "Median Hospital Profit Margins Falls to Zero," *Healthcare Financial Management* 63, no. 4 (April 2009): 18.
4. Damian Paletta, "Lending Declines as Bank Jitters Persist," *Wall Street Journal* (November 25, 2009): A10.
5. HFMA News, "Cost Concerns Lead to Healthcare Cutbacks," *Healthcare Financial Management* 63, no. 4 (April 2009): 18.
6. Anna Wilde Mathews, "CBO Chief Is Health-Care Referee," *Wall Street Journal* (April 21, 2008): A4.
7. Simona Covel, "Recession Batters Small Businesses, Threatening Owners' Dreams," *Wall Street Journal* (December 26, 2008): A8.
8. Thomas Friedman, "Into the Lean Years," *St. Petersburg Times* (February 23, 2010): 9A.
9. Joe Carlson and Melanie Evans, "No Brakes," *Modern Healthcare* (February 8, 2010): 6–7.
10. *USA Today*, "On Health Care, Republicans Move beyond 'Just Say No'" [editorial], *USA Today* (May 29, 2009): 6A.
11. Vanessa Fuhrmans, "Earnings Appear Unhealthy for Insurers," *Wall Street Journal* (April 21, 2008): B3.
12. Ibid.
13. Lawrence Rout, "Annual Checkup," *Wall Street Journal* (October 27, 2009): R2.
14. Carlson and Evans, "No Brakes," 6.
15. Steve Sternberg and Jack Gillum, "'Double Failure' at USA's Hospitals," *USA Today* (July 9, 2009): 1.
16. Marie McCullough and Josh Goldstein, "VA's Prostate Treatment Woes Began at Penn," *Philadelphia Inquirer* (August 9, 2009): 1, A15.
17. Joseph Pereira and Keith J. Winstein, "Benefit of Popular Spinal Surgery Is Questioned," *Wall Street Journal* (August 6, 2009): D1–D2.
18. Josh Goldstein, "5 Area Hospitals' Open-Heart Deaths Surprisingly High," *Philadelphia Inquirer* (August 6, 2009): 1, A15.
19. Jeffrey McCracken, "Mergers Thrive in Health Industry," *Wall Street Journal* (October 20, 2009): B1–B2.
20. Vincent Ciotti, principal, H.I.S. Professionals LLC, interview with author, Santa Fe, New Mexico, October 8, 2009.

21. David L. Bernd, CEO, Sentara Healthcare, interview with author, Norfolk, Virginia, October 13, 2009.
22. Ciotti interview.
23. Jacob Goldstein, "U.S. Hospitals Slow to Adopt E-Records," *Wall Street Journal* (March 26, 2009): A2.
24. Letitia Stein, "Enough Doctors to Go Around?" *St. Petersburg Times* (September 30, 2009): 1, 6A.
25. Herbert Pardes, "The Coming Shortage of Doctors," *Wall Street Journal* (November 5, 2009): A19.
26. Laura Landro, "For Severely Ill Children, a Dearth of Doctors," *Wall Street Journal* (January 12, 2010): D3.
27. HFMA News, "HFMA Releases Outlook Report," *Healthcare Financial Management* 63, no. 4 (April 2009): 30.
28. Joe Carlson, "Struggling with Shortages," *Modern Healthcare* (February 1, 2010): 10.
29. Holman W. Jenkins, Jr., "Why Obama Bombed on Health Care," *Wall Street Journal* (September 30, 2009): A21.
30. Richard Vodra, "The Next Energy Crises," *Financial Planning*, October 1, 2005 [http://www.financial-planning.com/news/next-energy-crisis-527174-1.html]. Accessed November 19, 2009.
31. Greater New Orleans Community Data Center.
32. Betsy McKay and Jennifer Corbett Dooren, "Vaccine Output Falls Short," *Wall Street Journal* (October 24, 2009): 1.
33. Jerry P. Widman, former chief financial officer, Ascension Health, interview with author, Dawsonville, Georgia, October 8, 2009.
34. Pardes, "The Coming Shortage," 30.
35. Douglas D. Hawthorne, president and CEO, Texas Health Resources, interview with author, Arlington, Texas, September 21, 2009.
36. Stephanie Strom, "Costly Charities," *Sunday News* (December 6, 2009): A1, A5.
37. Francis X. Ryan, president, Ryan and Associates Ltd., and former board chair, St. Agnes Hospital, interview with author, Lebanon, Pennsylvania, November 25, 2009.

A

State-by-State Summary of Merger Activity Comparing the 5-Year Merger Mania Period (1994–98) with the Succeeding 10 Years (1999–2008)

State	1994–98 (5 years)	1999–2008 (10 years)	Total (15 years)
Alabama	24	21	45
Alaska	1	1	2
Arizona	11	10	21
Arkansas	8	13	21
California	62	51	113
Colorado	5	3	8
Connecticut	7	2	9
Delaware	1	1	2
District of Columbia	1	6	7
Florida	47	29	76
Georgia	19	20	39
Hawaii	1	3	4
Idaho	3	3	6
Illinois	22	22	44
Indiana	15	32	47
Iowa	8	4	12
Kansas	9	5	14
Kentucky	9	11	20
Louisiana	15	27	42
Maryland	6	6	12
Massachusetts	31	7	38
Michigan	23	11	34
Minnesota	18	3	21
Mississippi	9	19	28
Missouri	20	11	31

State	1994–98 (5 years)	1999–2008 (10 years)	Total (15 years)
Montana	2	—	2
Nebraska	8	4	12
Nevada	3	2	5
New Hampshire	3	1	4
New Jersey	25	10	35
New Mexico	2	6	8
New York	47	20	67
North Carolina	16	12	28
North Dakota	5	5	10
Ohio	38	28	66
Oklahoma	16	16	32
Oregon	3	12	15
Pennsylvania	41	38	79
Rhode Island	5	—	5
South Carolina	16	3	19
South Dakota	1	3	4
Tennessee	20	30	50
Texas	61	50	111
Utah	10	2	12
Vermont	2	—	2
Virginia	12	18	30
Washington	4	4	8
West Virginia	10	11	21
Wisconsin	18	3	21
Wyoming	1	1	2
Total	**744**	**600**	**1,344**

Source: Author's compilation of data from *Modern Healthcare*'s *Annual Merger and Acquisition Report*, 1994 to 2008.

APPENDIX
B

States with the Most For-Profit Activity over a 15-Year Period, 1994–2008

State	1994–98 (5 years)	1999–2008 (10 years)	Total (15 years)
Texas	34	40	74
California	31	40	71
Florida	31	23	54
Alabama	14	27	41
Louisiana	12	25	37
Tennessee	11	20	31
Georgia	9	17	26
Oklahoma	9	14	23
Mississippi	8	14	22
Ohio	12	10	22
Illinois	8	12	20
Pennsylvania	3	16	19
Virginia	8	11	19
Totals	190	269	459

Source: Author's compilation from *Modern Healthcare*'s *Annual Merger and Acquisition Report*, 1994 to 2008.

For-profit activity comprises transactions with for-profits, with other for-profits, or with not-for-profits.

Excluded from the list are large, interstate health system mergers and acquisitions (see chapter 1 for highlights).

APPENDIX
C

Sample Physician Letters
Soliciting Voluntary Surcharge
Payments by Patients

XXX X. XXX, MD

Any Street
Any Town, Any State

December 2008

Dear Patient,

Once again I am making an appeal to you, my patient, to make a strictly voluntary surcharge payment of one hundred dollars ($100) so that I can maintain my medical practice. Through your past generosity I have been able to keep my practice going, despite rising expenses and decreasing revenues.

This year I am faced with the same dilemma of either changing the style of my general internal medicine primary care practice by using physician extenders such as nurse practitioners to see my patients, cutting back on my time spent with patients to increase volume, cutting back on personnel and office space, or continuing the style of practice that has worked so well over the past thirty-plus years I have been in practice.

With your continued help I will be able to maintain my current style of practice and the patient-doctor relationship that is needed to survive in this difficult health care situation we all find ourselves in at this time.

Please remember this $100 surcharge is strictly voluntary and will in no way affect our ongoing relationship. The current economic times are not easy, and I realize some of you are under financial stress, but to those who can donate the voluntary surcharge, I will be very appreciative.

Please sign the enclosed document and, if you so choose, send it along with your check for the voluntary surcharge payment to my office at your convenience.

Thank you.

Regards,

XXX X. XXX, MD

XXX X. XXX, MD

Any Street
Any Town, Any State

December 2008

Dear Patient,

Practice costs have risen out of sight in the past several years. Operating expenses far exceed current revenue. I will not be able to practice medicine, as you and I know it, without assistance from you, my wonderful patient. If you agree, I will continue to do my best.

Failure to agree will not be associated with any change in our current relationship.

Sincerely,

XXX X. XX, MD

The following is an acknowledgment that my insurance carrier and/or Medicare will not cover the needed surcharge expenses, and I voluntarily agree to one of the following options:

ANNUAL ($100)   _____
        OR
I will not support the surcharge.   _____

_____   _____
Signature   Date

_____
Please Print Name

Please respond and mail back to:
Dr. XXX X. XXX
Any Street
Any Town, Any State

Index